That Other Place

That Other Place

A PERSONAL ACCOUNT OF BREAST CANCER

Penelope Williams

Dundurn Press
Toronto and Oxford
1993

Copyright © Penelope Findlay Williams, 1993

All rights reserved. No part of this publication may be reproduced, stored in a retrieval system, or transmitted in any form or by any means, electronic, mechanical, photocopying, recording, or otherwise (except brief passages for purposes of review) without the prior permission of Dundurn Press Limited. Permission to photocopy should be requested from the Canadian Reprography Collective.

Printed and bound in Canada

The publisher wishes to acknowledge the generous assistance and ongoing support of **The Canada Council, The Book Publishing Industry Development Program** of the **Department of Communications, The Ontario Arts Council, The Ontario Publishing Centre** of the **Ministry of Culture, Tourism and Recreation,** and **The Ontario Heritage Foundation.**
Care has been taken to trace the ownership of copyright material used in the text. The author and publisher welcome any information enabling them to rectify any reference or credit in subsequent editions.

J. Kirk Howard, Publisher

Grateful acknowledgement is made to Faber and Faber Ltd. (London) for permission to reprint the excerpt from "Punishment," by Seamus Heaney, on pages 63–64.

Canadian Cataloguing in Publication Data

Williams, Penelope, 1943 –
    That other place: a personal account of breast cancer

Includes bibliographical references.
ISBN 1-55002-203-2 (paper)

1. Breast – Cancer. I. Title.

RC280.B8W5   1993   616.99'449'0092   C93–095350-9

Dundurn Press Limited
2181 Queen Street East
Suite 301
Toronto, Canada
M4E 1E5

Dundurn Distribution
73 Lime Walk
Headington, Oxford
England
0X3 7AD

Dundurn Press Limited
1823 Maryland Avenue
P.O. Box 1000
Niagara Falls, N.Y.
U.S.A. 14302-1000

Contents

Acknowledgements / ix

Foreword / xi

Prologue / xv

-I-
Crossing the Border / 1
-II-
BC/AD: New Meaning / 9
-III-
Myths and Shibboleths / 13
-IV-
Why Me? Well, Why Not Me? / 18
-V-
Simon Says, "Take One Giant Step ... FAST" / 25
-VI-
Just How Fatal Is It? / 33
-VII-
The Search for Better Odds / 37
-VIII-
Wrestling with Reality / 44
-IX-
Brief Encounter with the Technocrats / 51

Contents

-X-
Simon Says, "Take Another Giant Step: Chemotherapy" / 54

-XI-
Chemotherapy Fallout #1: Hair / 63

-XII-
Chemotherapy Fallout #2: Nausea, Up, Down and Sideways / 69

-XIII-
Only a Pause on the Journey / 79

-XIV-
Chemotherapy Fallout #3: Instant Menopause / 84

-XV-
The Simons Hold a Tumour Board Meeting / 95

-XVI-
The Third Giant Step: Radiation / 104

-XVII-
Skirmishes on the Medical Front / 109

-XVIII-
Doctor as God / 116

-XIX-
On and Off the Bandwagons / 129

-XX-
Is There a Cancer Personality? / 144

-XXI-
Taking Control / 151

-XXII-
Mind/Body Medicine: Dealing with the Guilt / 161

-XXIII-
Bernie Siegel: Peace, Love and Jokes / 171

Contents

-XXIV-
Clyve / 180

-XXV-
Mind Over Cancer / 188

-XXVI-
Every Little Thing Helps / 198

-XXVII-
Hollyhock / 206

-XXVIII-
The Dragon Slayers / 213

-XXIX-
Dragon at the Door / 217

-XXX-
Be Glad You Have Cancer …? / 222

Selected Bibliography / 231

To my sons, Matt and Sam
To my husband, Allen

Acknowledgements

Acknowledgements — such a bland word to describe a wealth of gratitude. This whole book is an acknowledgement to the many people who brought me through the dark years of diagnosis, illness and treatment and back into a new life where the spectre of breast cancer, instead of striding about centre stage, skulks now in a muffled, offstage corner.

To Dr. Diane Twemlow, Dr. C.D. Chadwick and Dr. Susan Aitken for being such good medical guides in "that other place."

To friends in both places: Andy Spry and Lucy McCormick who kept me sane with their friendship and laughter on chemo days; Bron Westerman and Elly McCrea whose visits bridged the years and an ocean; and those friends I travelled with in the new world, so many of whom are gone now. They appear throughout this book but usually under another name to protect their privacy.

To Sylvia Rosenes, a companion in both worlds, who said just before she died, "If I am in your book, use my real name. And try to tell people how to leave, OK?" Her first request, I could fulfil, but not her second.

To Rex Williams, Judy Steed and Tim Plumptre, who had faith enough in both my writing and my survival abilities to support my application to the Canada Council Explorations Program. And to Dr. Balfour Mount, a stranger whose kind support was incentive for me to persevere even when the words would not come.

To the Canada Council for awarding me a grant through the Explorations Program.

Acknowledgements

To my family, Seaton and Sue Findlay, Mobe and Joan Findlay and all their kids; to Dad; and to my "steps," Loranne, Patrick, Keith, Jennifer, Shannon and Allen, Jr., all who, in the early black months, leaned through the windows to help tighten the ropes around the dragon.

To my husband Allen Sackmann, and my sons, Matt and Sam, without whom this book would not have been written ... because without them I would not have been around long enough to write it.

Penelope Williams
1993

Foreword

The only thing predictable about breast cancer is that it is unpredictable. Where it strikes, and whom, its speed of growth, remissions and response to treatment are all wild cards. All the oncologists, surgeons, chemo nurses, radiologists and psychologists I have encountered eventually say the same thing, as they clamber about on the crumbling, shifting cliff of cancer data. To keep from slipping right off into the unknown, they use statistics, the toe clamps and climbing axes of their profession.

Why do some people get cancer, and others in the same family, sharing the same genes, the same environment, the same diet, don't? Why do some people conquer the disease, and others apparently succumb so quickly, whatever the treatment? Why is breast cancer so prevalent in North America and not in Japan? Why do some patients suffer debilitating side-effects from exactly the same chemotherapy and radiation regimens taken by others who sail through treatment relatively unscathed. Why has there been so little progress in finding a cure?

And why has this been the same story for *more than 25 years?*

> [S]o little has really changed in the history of treating breast cancer, that 25 years after my mother was diagnosed with cancer I am far more advanced in my disease than she was. Two women a century apart, diagnosed with single tumours the same size, neither of which showed any signs of spread, yet we have different stories to tell. She is alive and apparently free and clear of the disease. I, on the other hand, am literally fighting for my life with metastases in my lungs, bones and liver. (*Breast Cancer: Unanswered Questions*, p. 4)

Foreword

Individual responses to the diagnosis, the disease and the treatment are medically legion; it seems the ravages and retreats of the disease are monstrous and arbitrary.

However, a core of common experience does provide a foundation for research; these common elements are the building blocks of statistics and the touchstones for cancer sufferers casting about for the comfort a shared understanding provides.

To know of others whose experience is similar to yours strikes a comforting chord: you are not completely out of tune with the rest of humanity after all.

∞

This book is in the nature of a travelogue: reports filed from my journey in the world of breast cancer. After diagnosis and surgery, the first two steps on this journey which happened in jig time within blurred days of each other, I went through a schizophrenic period of reading everything available on the subject of breast cancer, at the same time determined not to take in a single word in case it told me what I didn't want to hear. My need to know was fanatical, a desperate scratching for crumbs that would reassure. I wanted to learn about other people with breast cancer in Canada, close to home, people whose experience might reflect mine a little.

In my peeled and raw state, actual conversations on the subject were too threatening. The printed word offered a semblance of control in a world where I had completely lost it; I could slam the book shut before some destructive but "research-proven" fact or loopy, off-the-wall fiction crept into my consciousness. Tempered judgements were among the first casualties of the cancer diagnosis grenade. Later they would rise shakily from the debris and start sifting through the craziness of fact and myth I was collecting.

But before venturing beyond the privacy of books, articles and videos, I had to come to terms with the realization that I had cancer, a disease that only other people had.

After the terror of diagnosis, the shuddering fear of surgery and what more might be found, came the black, paralysing depression that shut down the runways of my brain like fog at an airport. The information I thought I was seeking never landed. At the beginning, I reeled and bumped off meaningless paragraphs, and the teetering stack of books on cancer gathered dust by my bed. In the end, who cared; none of this was going to help me. It was all words, mostly words from Britain or the United States, or from doctors who talked from the safe side of the subject. My brain went into hibernation that felt like terminal dormancy.

Slowly, though, I moved back to wanting to know more, this time a saner, more controlled desire for knowledge and support. Now I was more willing to talk to people about it, therapists, other cancer sufferers (or, in the cancer lingo, "survivors"). Doors started opening in this claustrophobic country.

Fear, anger, laughter, despair — the stories of other cancer sufferers helped validate my own feelings; these shared experiences had one message, "You are not alone in this mess." Well, of course I was; we all are. That aloneness is ultimately the human condition intensified through the isolation of a life-threatening illness. At the same time, though, we are busily denying our island status. Shared experiences make one of the most important bridges. The resulting empathy and understanding among travellers in this barren land are as important to healing as are all the medical treatments.

Time and again in the last five years I have heard the same feelings expressed: "What a relief to talk to someone else who has cancer. I don't have to explain, I don't have to justify, I don't have to pretend ..." I have felt that too. It isn't a fellowship of our choosing but it is a bond that softens the pain of a journey in "that other place."

Illness is the night-side of life, a more onerous citizenship. Everyone who is born holds dual citizenship, in the kingdom of the well and in the kingdom of the sick. Although we all prefer to use only the good passport, sooner or later each of us is obliged, at least for a spell, to identify ourselves as citizens of that other place.

Susan Sontag
Illness as Metaphor

Prologue

A Friday evening in late April, school over for the week, work put aside until Monday. The western sky flowed with the liquid light of spring, bathing the earth in a brief, aching brilliance before dark. We — my husband, Allen, and my two sons, Matt and Sam — sat at the dinner table, chatting, idling, watching the wheeling flocks of birds over the back yard. The boys told school stories and argued mildly over whose turn it was to do the dishes.

As it was still too cool to linger on the deck, Allen and I sat just inside the patio doors, drinking the last of our wine, welcoming spring, making plans.

When the phone rang, neither of us moved. It would be for one of the boys, weekend schemes to hatch.

"For you, Mum," Matt handed me the phone. "I think it's Sylvia."

Sylvia, a good friend, a funny lady — her conversations laced with wit. But not this night. She was in hospital, she'd had the operation, it didn't look good. She chose her words carefully, weaving phrases and courage into a cloak to soften the message. It was cancer...

The sky was bled of light now, and with the dark came back the winter cold. I pulled the curtains against the night and the muffled footfalls of the dragon that had slouched into our lives.

-1-
Crossing the Border

Does the road wind uphill all the way?
Yes, to the very end.
Will the day's journey take the whole long day?
From morn to night, my friend.
    Christina Georgina Rossetti, *Uphill*

In Canada, one in nine women will be diagnosed with breast cancer. That represents 14,400 new cases this year; that represents more than 10 percent of the female population; that represents too many. Unlike some other cancers, incidence rates are not declining, in fact the opposite: epidemiologists say that breast cancer is very much on the increase, about one percent a year since 1964.

Epidemiology, the study of causes of disease, derives from the same root as the word "epidemic." In 1989, in Ontario alone 4,000 women were diagnosed with breast cancer; 304 individuals were diagnosed with AIDS. The onslaught of AIDS is being described as an epidemic. In the last 12 months, 10,000 people have died of cholera in South and Central America. The recurrence of cholera in such numbers is referred to as an epidemic. Epidemiologists estimate that 5,100 women will die of breast cancer this year ... *in one country, Canada*. (All the statistics on the incidence of breast cancer are taken from the parliamentary sub-committee report, *Breast Cancer: Unanswered Questions*.) It is not outrageous to suggest that, despite the fact that breast cancer is not contagious, what we are dealing with here is an epidemic.

That Other Place

One in nine, one in 10, one in 20 is one too many. One in any number is too many, especially if you are that one.

In September 1988 I fell onto the wrong side of this statistical equation: instead of being unthinkingly one of eight, I became unthinkably the one in nine.

My itinerary from hell began when the results of a second needle biopsy contradicted a mammogram and a first biopsy six weeks earlier. But that might not have been Day 1 on this journey. It could have been Day 14 or Day 600 or even Day 24,000 depending on what theory you believe. Cancer can be quietly incubating for up to 20 years, according to some oncological researchers, and the silent, or incubation, period before there is any lump at all "is considerably longer than the period we do know a tumor is present." (Dollinger *et al.*, p. 2) The smallest detectable malignant lump in the breast — about one centimetre — already contains one billion cancer cells. (*Ibid.*, p. 244)

During my first weeks in this new and hostile land, I clutched at one theory after another with fevered desperation in the search for why I was on this journey at all. What started the cancer in me? Was it stress, environment, diet, a passing germ, or had it been lying dormant in the genes of my forebears?

Most people remember exactly the details of the day of their diagnosis, the day the travel plans they never made are confirmed. Each tiny detail is bathed in the harsh light of shock, of fear and bewilderment. And at departure time, the medical community provides most of us with a travel guide. Not everyone is so lucky. One woman I met was flung out of her comfortable world with a telephone call and not even a bon voyage from her doctor. "Marjorie? The test results are positive," this medical paragon spoke into the phone. "You have a malignant brain tumour. Unfortunately it is only stage one which means we can't treat it until it gets bigger. My office will be in touch in a few months."

Goodbye. Have a nice day, you and your tiny new brain tumour.

Most people have more warning — perhaps symptoms that have plagued them for years — so that when diagnosis comes, it is confirmation of already lurking suspicions. How ever you begin, your life is rent in two by that word "cancer" trailing its associations of pain, hopelessness and death. Suddenly BC and AD take on new meaning: Before Cancer and After Diagnosis.

The lump I found in my breast was a tiny little thing that squirmed away and seemed to disappear under my touch. Atavistic apprehension that surely every women feels at even the thought of a breast lump, and the admonitions of recent magazine articles on breast cancer, sent me off to my doctor. Fast. It was she who saved me from the false reassurances of medical science — a Human outwitting the Machine. I would have continued for God knows how long, temporarily intact but festering toward self-destruct, before the much-touted, early warning tools caught up with her instinct.

"I am almost certain it is OK," she said, rolling the offending morsel like a piece of dough between her fingers, "but you should go for a mammogram anyway."

The X-ray not only revealed nothing suspicious — it didn't even reveal the lump we knew was there. This was not exactly a convincing demonstration of the efficacy of mammograms.

"Hmm. I don't think you need to worry," my GP said, "but I'd like a second opinion anyway. I'm referring you to a surgeon who specializes in breast ..." She did not finish the phrase, "breast cancer." Apparently this surgeon just specialized in breasts. "I'll track the lump for a month until he can see you. He'll probably scoff and send you home, but never mind."

He did not quite scoff and send me home but was as "almost certain" as my GP. A tall, youngish, round-eyed man, with a Mr. Hulot walk, he made me feel that all small breakables in his vicinity should be nailed down. Despite his windmill tendencies, and his later constant admonitions to "stay cool" while his eyes signalled such anguish, I liked him. More important, I trusted him. That trust was to be a lifeline.

After poking and prodding me, he declared that it was the size of a frozen pea. I reared up from the examination table, indignant.

"The lump, I mean the lump," he said hastily. "Hey, I'm 99 percent sure that it is benign, almost certain there is nothing to worry about. It is separate. There is no suppuration from the nipple; it just feels OK. But we'll do a needle biopsy just to be positive."

He jabbed a needle into the lump, peeled me off the ceiling and sent me on my way to wait for the results of the test on the cells that he had extracted.

Within three days his nurse phoned to give me the all clear. Whoopee. Off the hook. Of course I knew that would be the result. Cancer only happens to other people. Armed with the negative findings of a mammogram, a biopsy and two doctors, I could forget the whole business. Well, not quite. I was to go back in six weeks and if the lump was still there, the surgeon would remove it. Just a tiny operation, local anaesthetic, in and out of hospital the same day.

About then I made my first mistake. Or maybe it was a long line of mistakes and this was the final straw for the gods who sit up there somewhere pulling wings off flies. I said, *out loud*, right where anyone could hear, when quizzed by my 13-year-old son, Sam, "No, love, don't worry, I don't have breast cancer."

Well, I might as well have stood up in a boat in the middle of the lake and shouted at those gods to strike me with lightning if they were listening. Gods have very acute hearing.

At the end of the summer I went back for the check-up. The lump was indeed still there, no bigger, just a miniature hand grenade with its pin pulled, leaking its billion cancer cells. When I told Mr. Hulot, the surgeon, that it seemed to ache now, his eyes lit up, he flung out his arm expansively, and dove for the pile of papers he had swept from his desk.

"Great, that means it's probably a cyst. Let's see if we can get some fluid off that sucker."

I was beginning to feel like a regular on that ceiling of his.

"Nope, it's a solid little bugger. Can't get a drop," he said, after what seemed to be about a day and a half of jabbing about. "Oh well, since I've put you through all this again, I might as well send these cells off to be checked. To be on the safe side."

I was to wonder what it must be like to be on that safe side.

Crossing the Border

∞

We were in the final preparations for a family dinner party in honour of a nephew's impending marriage, an activity only slightly less hectic than a NASA launching — the party, not the marriage. Sue, my sister-in-law and good friend, and I had been meeting for lunch for weeks to discuss menus, guest lists, seating plans, and talking about everything but. The morning of the dinner, we were organizing Sue's dining-room, trying to figure out a way of seating 22 people at a table for 12. This took many cups of coffee and several bits of paper with indecipherable scribbles.

"Why can't we have a buffet?" her son, John, asked absently, picking out a tune on his guitar.

He pronounced "buffet" as if it were a high wind on a mountain top, an often apt description of our family parties. They swirl with chat, argument, laughter. All the world's problems are resolved around our dinner tables, at decibels that would crack glass. Three generations of opinions, jokes, debates, family anecdotes; bets and counter-bets on who wrote what book, where is that quotation from, who is a Good Writer, who a Bad One, why and ... wait, wait, what about, no listen, that can't be right, it was *Butch Cassidy*, not *The Sting* ... Betch ya a dinner at Al's ... You're on. Always another book to discuss, a film to dissect, another weekend to plan or point to make, another gust of laughter. These parties were truly buffets.

"Because a buffet isn't elegant enough for tonight. This is going to be a truly swank affair." Sue swung a foot up on a chair, leaned on her knee and squinted through a curl of cigarette smoke down the table, which looked like a highway after the spring frost heaves. It was certainly not elegant. We had extended the dining-room table with a card table, an ironing board and a rickety desk with legs like snares. A 20-foot tablecloth was to hide all sins. Except that it was still at the cleaners from the last party.

"Not only will this party start elegant. It'll end elegant," I remarked from the vantage point of the doorway, since I couldn't get any further into the room.

That Other Place

"Why so?"

"Because everyone will be so squished in, they won't be able to get their arms out to eat. The pristine beauty of our table will remain intact forever."

"Miss Haversham, eat your heart out."

"I still don't see why we can't do buffet," John spoke between chords, his blond head bent over his guitar.

"Because all you kids will go down to the rec room with your plates. The adults'll head for the den, and Gramps will haul a chair up to the table regardless and we'll all have to eddy around him like a snag in the rapids," I answered.

"Like what?"

"A snag. A snag."

"Is this a stag?" John strummed a fancy intro: "Her name is Patricia, *strumm*. She calls herself Delicia, *strumm*. And she's the best damn stripper in towwwn."

"Benches, that's what we need," Sue dropped her foot to the floor with decision. "Then we can get everyone in. It's the chairs that take up all the room. Where will we get benches?"

We had two on our deck, and I went home for them. It was a familiar well-trodden route between our houses, only a few blocks apart. It went past the elementary school where John, his sister, Nic, and my Matt had gone. Although he didn't attend the school, Sam certainly had a place in its mythology by virtue of the stone he pegged through a window, an action he owned up to in a note that earned him public praise over the school's announcements the following day.

The route included the sidewalks where my brother walked his dog every morning, carrying a little plastic bag of what I'm sure was permanent dog poop to fool the Neighbourhood Watch. Around the corner, under a canopy of maple trees and down half a block to our house, it's a walk I've done a thousand times, early mornings with the dogs, afternoons for a cup of coffee and a chat, late in the darkness after communal dinners or parties. It was a route that sometimes took a minute, sometimes hours as the night we all lay on the dew-drenched grass and watched the northern lights until dawn.

Crossing the Border

The message light on the telephone answering machine was flashing. I punched the replay absently, hoping there were no urgent business calls because I wanted to take the whole day off.

"This is Dr. _____'s office. Could you please call as soon as possible?"

Geez. The second biopsy. I had almost forgotten about it.

Dialling the number, I was only mildly anxious, my mind on more important things such as where were the silver serving bowls.

"Mrs. Williams? The doctor tried to reach you earlier. He'd like to see you tomorrow at one o'clock."

"Why? What's wrong?" I could hear my voice asking the question, but suddenly this was not happening to me. It was not my voice, it was not my life.

"Something is not quite right. He wants to talk to you about your last test." The nurse gave nothing away, her white-uniformed voice cool and without nuance.

The gods had hurled their lightning bolt, slapping their knees and chortling. Is there life after lightning? Scorched senseless, it was months before I could look beyond each dragging step to find out.

Back at Sue's I went through the motions of setting the table, writing out menus, folding napkins. But I had already left my secure, familiar world where events happened as planned, where I could organize a family party and know I'd be there, a world unmindful of the banana peel around the corner. I had been rocketed into a new country, and already the old one was receding.

Looking back, I see that summer and early autumn in an idyllic glow that hindsight bathes the innocent days before a cataclysm. In my more pretentious moments, when I was practising to put Me First, as all the "heal-yourself" gurus instructed, that time held only slightly less portent than the hot, unsuspecting summer of 1914 before World War I.

Perspective is one of the first casualties of cancer. Mine staggered along with me through the days of my journey, swinging

That Other Place

me on and off bandwagons, in and out of terror; my slightly demented travelling companion never completely abandoned or misled me, but it certainly gave me some bad moments.

-II-
BC/AD: *New Meaning*

It is not quite the same journey from the cradle to the grave each time. Sometimes the differences are small, sometimes they are very important. We must set out each time on the same road but along that road we have a choice of adventures.

J.B. Priestley, *I Have Been Here Before*

The pathological report had identified "suspicious cells." Mr. Hulot described the findings to Allen and me, what they meant and what the next steps would be. He was thorough, he even drew a diagram. I understood nothing except that I would have surgery in less than a week to take out the lump, the surrounding tissue, which as far as I knew could mean everything between my neck and my kneecap, and some lymph nodes under my arm. What were lymph nodes? No idea. Whatever they were, they would be sent for examination and the results would indicate if and how far the cancer had spread. Hard to believe now that I could have been so unaware of these little items, like knots in a rope, used to calibrate a patient's statistical likelihood of survival. I grew to see them as miniature cesspools of cancer lurking in the recesses of what was left of my armpit.

Mr. Hulot was "almost certain" that they would test negative. He was equally "almost certain" that indeed the lump was malignant. Only a two percent chance that the last test was wrong.

"Now don't worry, don't worry, don't worry. It won't do any good. Stay cool. Stay cool." He looked frantically around for

That Other Place

escape from the pain of this conversation. Later, I wondered how I was so trusting of a surgeon whose physical presence threatened all inanimate objects. Perhaps that was his secret. He wasn't operating on an inanimate object. He was carving up a human being, and his sensitivity and connection with his patients translated into the magic skill of his hands. But not to his words of helpless reassurance. Stay cool? Would frozen stiff do? If I were any cooler I'd be dead. And Allen was an iceberg.

The creeping paralysis of euphemisms had begun with "something not quite right" to "something wrong" to "suspicious cells" to "malignant cells," tiny malevolent creatures, evil, slimy, legions of them with minuscule hoods and machine guns loaded with poison, slithering down in platoons out of the tumour, across my shoulder and into the lymph system, taking each node as an occupying army destroys a village in its path. Such feverish images came later.

Mr. Hulot apparently could not bring himself to say, "You have breast cancer." He circled the statement, darting in and out and around it, but I don't believe he ever actually said it then, not that first visit.

Such terms as "invading ductal carcinoma" did pop up in the conversation — I have this in my notes but not in my memory. My brain had closed down, blocking great chunks of the discussion. I remember hearing the suppressed and helpless rage in Allen's voice as he asked questions. Here was a situation that all his strength of purpose was not going to be able to bring under control. A resourceful and determined man, he was to show me later how he dealt with this invasion — by replacing wishes with prayer.

The Chinese water torture of ever more specific jargon leading up to the actual word CANCER had reduced me to complete inertia. Slowly, slowly, in waves crashing and receding, the realization cloudily took hold that I had cancer. I could see myself as if at the end of a long tunnel, distant and healthy and glowing at the other end. The old me, so far away already.

My old world, the world I had so taken for granted, was gone. No time for a Wolfian journey of the soul, no time for leisurely lessons and recognitions: the knowledge that I couldn't go home again was especially jolting since I hadn't even known I'd left.

Like zombies, we left the surgeon's office. We got in the car, and we drove.

Allen wanted to go up to the chalet we were starting to build at Grand Lake, a few miles from Ottawa, our dream house that had been on the drawing board for years. We had designed and redesigned it a hundred times, even tracing its floor plan to full scale in the sand floor of a local gravel pit. As I had done in the leaf houses of my childhood, we stepped over the lines in the sand from room to room, the finished house vivid in our imaginations. A whole winter of evenings was strewn with our graph paper layouts for windows, decks, cosy and lofty spaces to house our future. The foundation, the real one, had been dug just a month earlier.

I wanted to go to the family cottage, a few miles beyond Aylmer on the Quebec side of the Ottawa River, a big rambling turn-of-the-century place built by my grandfather. I didn't want to go the chalet because it was the future and I didn't seem to have one anymore.

The "Aimers" drew me with its security of the past. It is a place redolent of childhood summers, days my father called "Sweet Do-Nothing Time":

Now the world is set at idle,
Summer at its prime
With the high white-clouded weather
And Sweet Do-Nothing Time.

Nothing much happened, and everything happened in those lazy summers echoing with the generations of children before us. The cicadas — or the tree frogs or the hydro wires, depending on who was doing the explaining — pierced the shimmering heat with their metallic twang; we argued lazily about whether it was too hot to play badminton; we swam; we caught fireflies in the twilight, letting them go before they blinked out for good.

That Other Place

We dared explore the woods behind the cottage in the velvet dark, half out of our minds with delicious terror. When the fear became too real we raced back to the haven of the verandah and the grown-ups.

The most threatening events were the sudden storms that thundered down the wide expanse of river, lightning hissing into the water. When the first blast of wind sent the trees thrashing around the cottage and the shredded curtains of rain roared across the water, only then would we scamper for shelter from the storm.

The Aimers still throngs with family, alive and dead. The verandah screen door slams as it has done for 90 years of children racing through; at the end of day, the western sun slants in under the porch roof on everyone gathered for late afternoon tea, a ritual that has lasted nearly a century.

Like an X-ray, the sun bounces off the glittering lake and the burnt grass of the front lawn. Someone lowers the tangled green slatted blind, and the sudden cool envelops the verandah group stunned into silence by the heat. That's when the other voices can be heard, the voices of family gone before — my sister, my Mum, her sisters and brothers, their parents, they are all there, the most unthreatening of ghosts, watching over us all.

I was running for shelter now, from the storm blast of diagnosis, from the relentless terror of what I could only guess was in store for me. There, in the old cottage, I would be safe again, deep in the heart of my family that had always protected me before.

That day, Allen and I drove sort of in the direction of the cottage but we had lost our compass. Neither of us had the will to reach any destination. We drove around and round, trapped in the present, up and down streets, trying to get away rather than to arrive.

-III-
Myths and Shibboleths

Is not disease the rule of existence?

Henry David Thoreau, *Journal,* 1851

Cancer's arsenal of destruction includes not just the cells that run amok in the physical body; much of its power lies in its mythology and reputation, hardened over centuries into a carapace of dread. It has a deservedly bad press. Its only admirers are those few self-deluded intimates who, desperate in its sickening embrace, declaim that they needed it to focus them, to get their lives on the right track — the "every cloud has a silver lining" attitude stretched to absurdity.

Cancer carries with it the baggage of terror and despair of generations. As early as 1528, Thomas Paynell described cancer as "'a melancholye impostume, eatynge partes of the bodye ...' The very name — from the Greek *karkinos* and the Latin *cancer* both meaning crab — was inspired according to Galen, by the resemblance of an external tumour's veins to a crab's legs." (Sontag, p. 10) It is a spectre throughout literature and lore, the dark, stark image stalking the sunlit lives of the unsuspecting. And when it strikes, despite 20th-century medicine and new theories, the death knell is its signature tune, no matter the circumstances of the diagnosis.

Since cancer begins as an invisible disease, eroding the body from inside, it is generally depicted as a silent malevolence, an internal bubble of suppurating evil. By the time it reaches the outside of the body it is often too late, although its manifestations are usually portrayed as sudden and horrific — the skeletal wasted body, the mutant lumps and crazy growth of cells gone mad. And what ravages the disease doesn't cause, the treatments apparently do — the tufty bald skulls and streaming eyes of chemotherapy, the burnt and bleeding skin of radiation.

All these associations and images terrify, because, as the song says, there ain't no cure. You can't go to the doctor and get a vaccine to protect you from cancer. You can't take a few days off work while an antibiotic does its work. The "magic bullet" that Paul Ehrlich came up with as a treatment for syphilis in 1910 has not yet been found for breast cancer. There is the Salk serum for polio, insulin for diabetes and penicillin for TB. For breast cancer there is still only the buckshot approach: try everything — chronologically, in tandem, the whole shooting match — using statistics as the sighting aid. The "cure" is elusive as ever despite daily newspaper headlines to the contrary.

Cancer is used as the ultimate comparison, although now it is being given a run for its money by AIDS, the next disease in the line of plagues that keep the human race in check. But AIDS has anticipated its cue and has rushed on stage shouldering cancer out of the research limelight if not out of people's lives. Unfortunately though, they are not mutually exclusive. The very opposite, since AIDS weakens the immune system, throwing open the body's ramparts to terminal illness such as cancer.

Unlike the more orderly progression of bogeyman diseases that have prowled the centuries, AIDS has not waited its turn. Previous afflictions lingered and festered quietly until the one before it was conquered by medical science. In the Western world, tuberculosis was the killer in the early part of this century. Cancer certainly was around, possibly under the guise of a lot of other names as well as its own, but it didn't become the disease of the month until tuberculosis was almost eradicated with the discovery of antibiotics. Same with polio, with small pox, with cholera (at least in North America).

But cancer is still at the top of the dread charts. Renate Rubinstein, a Dutch journalist, writes about her struggle with multiple sclerosis in a fine book ... for everyone except readers with cancer. A relentless refrain runs through her prose, one that obviously gives her solace: "All my experience with illness has been that it goes away, except cancer," she writes. (p. 19) "[B]efore I became ill, I took it for granted, as do most people, that in our age a good doctor can cure anything, so long as it's not cancer." (p. 25) And: "Multiple sclerosis differs from cancer in that you can grow old with it." (p. 25) Yup, things are bad, very bad, but at least I don't have cancer.

The iteration flicked me into muttering at the pages as I read, "Yah, well at least I don't have MS. So Yah Na Na Na Na Nah."

But there you are — cancer is the final touchstone. Comfort me with cancer — the fact that I don't have it. So what about the rest of us, huddled in this other country, what touchstones do we have? Well, we have each other, and we have laughter, and we have an odd twisted satisfaction in the nighttime hours that we don't have to worry about getting cancer because we already have it. Which is short-lived comfort, since the biggest risk of all with breast cancer is whether you have had it before. All these comforts are of the Pollyanna sort anyway, tinsel touchstones that wither in the daylight.

Then there are the shibboleths of this other place — the common coin of cancer which undermines common sense, hope and the carefully angled blinkers against the close-up leer of cancer's visage. It helps to exorcise these destructive "facts" before they do you as much harm as the disease itself.

"Cancer is always fatal." So is life. As Peter Gzowski said to Stuart McLean one day on CBC's "Morningside": "People keep telling me the death rate is going up. But as far as I can see, it hasn't changed. It's still 100 percent. That is one statistic you can't argue with."

"Cancer is contagious." It's beginning to seem so because there is so much of it around. It might give every appearance of an epidemic, but it does not race through houses like the Black Death. It strikes like a great white shark, arrowing through a splashing crowd of swimmers to snatch one in an apparent random choice. Great whites are not contagious. Only unpredictable. So is cancer. That is a certainty, not a surmise.

"Cancer is shameful." Only in the eye of the beholder. It probably achieved this status because it starts invisibly, like an inner rot, and its use as metaphor for the horrific sustains its shameful reputation.

"Cancer is evil. It is God's way of punishing sinners." I don't believe in that kind of God. My faith is in a different God, benign, loving and perhaps sad at human ways, a faith strengthened by the incredible support and caring of the pastor, his wife and the congregation of Allen's church who scooped me up in love and prayer throughout my whole journey and still.

"Cancer is caused by other injuries." I don't want to believe this. Since Blitski, the clinical trial demon I encountered at the beginning of chemotherapy, expounded this theory, it has lost all credence for me (see chapter 9). I can't believe anything he said. That would be giving up a large chunk of sanity.

"We already have a cure for cancer; it's being tested now. It will be available very soon." I wish. Unfortunately, we read this statement practically every week. The follow-through is sadly lacking.

"If you have cancer, you can cure yourself." Guilt city. A dangerous shorthand that distorts by leaving out so much.

"You can leave everything to your doctors. They are the experts and they always know best." Uh huh. And if the experts disagree? Right there in front of you? Which one knows best?

"Caught early enough, cancer is curable." True and false. If you make it to five years, you are cured. Or three years. Or 16 years. This is statistical semantics, pure and simple.

"People with cancer have to be normal as soon as possible."

We would like to be, certainly. First of all though, what is "normal"? The old status quo, which may have been one of the factors that led to you getting cancer in the first place? And second, racing back to "normality" can induce such stress and guilt about not getting there quick enough, you simply get sick again.

"People who get cancer are passive, weak, out of touch with their own feelings, unable to express anger …" or "People who get cancer are angry, incapable of dealing with stress, depression, recent loss …" This is the cancer personality theory

Myths and Shibboleths

(see chapter 20 following). There perhaps is enough truth in some of this to make it harder to dismiss. So, like Samuel Johnson's irritable response to Berkeley's philosophy on reality, I am giving the table leg of this theory an almighty kick, muttering at the same time, "Thus I refute it."

A few of these myths have been paraphrased from Jacqueline Johnson's book, *Intimacy*. Some are ones I encountered first hand. They are all dangerous. The reputation, the myths and half-truths that festoon this disease are part of cancer's killing fields. They nail hope. They lock your brain into a paralysis while fear runs rampant. In the beginning. The only way to stay sane is to choose your own way, reduce panic by slamming doors on the most outrageous theories, choose the ones that you are most comfortable with and will yourself to have confidence in them. Easy to say.

-IV-
Why Me? Well, Why Not Me?

*Life is what happens to you
While you're busy
Making other plans*

John Lennon

The biggest struggle that first week had nothing to do with cancer theories, myths, cures or lies. It was straight damage control, trying to suppress terror and retain a veneer of normalcy with which to coat the days. One shaky day at a time. The nights were something else, loud with the wails of "Why me? Why me?" Anger, panic, despair and resentment took turns being tangible.

Allen also struggled with demons, his and mine. Like me, he admitted to a surging resentment at all the apparently healthy women who thronged his world — women who walked through his office building, women in front of him on the street, the women sitting on the porches that day we drove aimlessly up and down streets to nowhere. Why were all these women healthy, and suddenly now, not his own wife?

I had felt a degree of this kind of numb disbelief when John Kennedy was shot. From my room in university residence I had gazed down at the people walking in the driveway below, marvelling angrily that they could continue on as if nothing had happened. Hadn't the whole world changed with those rifle shots? Hadn't the whole world changed because I had cancer?

Why Me? Well, Why Not Me?

The short answer is no. The minor slings and arrows of ordinary life certainly didn't abate because a major one had hit the bull's-eye. For instance, I still got parking tickets.

Outraged, I wanted to race after the Green Hornet who buzzed happily down the row of cars, scattering tickets like pollen.

"A ticket! You can't give me a damn parking ticket! You can't bloody do that. I've got CANCER!"

His answer, if he had been an honest hornet, would have been "So what?" Cancer is not an antidote to bee stings.

Later I revised my thinking about those enviable paragons of good health. If even half the stories were true that people told me when they heard that I had cancer, these women were in fact sisters-in-law, all of whom without exception had recovered completely from a recent bout with breast cancer. (Not "of," but "with." You have a bout *of* flu, you have a bout *with* cancer — I guess because you must fight so hard with it; you can't just go to bed with a good book and a hot toddy until it runs its course.) For a while there no one ever died of cancer. You'd wonder what all the fuss was about, the way all these sisters-in-law shrugged it off.

"My sister-in-law had cancer," I was told so often in those early days. "She found a lump as big as an orange, and after it was removed, she had chemotherapy. She did lose all her hair, and she had a tough time taking care of her two small kids, but she's finished treatment now, and she looks wonderful, better than she's ever looked. And let's see, that was two years ago (or five years ago; one was even 35 years ago)."

"I just heard you were in hospital, Penny. A bad time for you. But listen, my sister-in-law had exactly the same thing. Two days before Christmas she went in for emergency surgery. She had chemotherapy for six months and was really mad because all her hair fell out except on her legs. She had to shave her legs through the whole treatment, and there she was bald as a tick. But she is fine now. Completely well."

These stories were meant to encourage, and they did. But I had to suspend disbelief in the face of such unrelentingly healthy sisters-in-law.

The most heartening account was about one who, at age 35, was diagnosed with a rare and fairly hefty cancer — one of the 100 or 150 variations. She had "aggressive treatment" and is well now. She had been severely ill with the same cancer as a teenager but it had been misdiagnosed then. If it been diagnosed correctly, she would have been told that it was immediately fatal since there was no way to treat it. By the time the doctors had figured out what it was, 17 years later, a treatment had been discovered.

It is conceivable that had she been told, the first time around, that she had an incurable cancer, she would have died. Such is the power of suggestion, of self-programming. Because she wasn't told, she didn't know, and proceeded to live happily for several more years until medical science caught up with her. Her recurrence coincided with the discovery of an effective treatment.

You think I was being fed skewed statistics, maybe? Not one story told to me in those early days featured a sister-in-law who, instead of being rosy and healthy after seven years, was pale and dead after one. A certain amount of censorship was at play here, because if everyone is so healthy after having cancer, why does the very word curdle your brain, why do people avert their eyes, avoid the subject and rush like nature into a vacuum to tell you about their amazingly healthy sisters-in-law?

However, this pattern imperceptibly changed and soon I was longing to hear about those vibrant creatures again. As people grew used to my illness, other stories started emerging. It was almost as if, since I appeared to be surviving relatively unscathed after surgery and a couple of months of chemotherapy, I had better not be allowed to be too cocky about it. A very few people seemed to want to let me know that there was a reality I might not be aware of — the distinct possibility that cancer might kill me.

After telling me about a close relative who was in hospital fighting her own brand of cancer with, so far, three different combinations of drugs, all unsuccessful, one friend said to me cheerfully, "And tonight we have to go to a wake for a friend, our age, who just died of intestinal cancer. It's really all around us, isn't it? Everywhere you turn."

Uh ... helloooo? Try *in* some of us, no matter where we turn.

On the days when self-pity was not completely rampant, I understood that the people with the bad-news stories were using me as a touchstone. There but for the grace of God go I, they were saying. I was making people feel better because they weren't me. That is a hell of role to find yourself in.

The "why me?" stage came and went for the first few months of treatment, manifesting itself sometimes in anger, sometimes in despair. Anger was healthier.

Each is one of the five stages of dying, identified by Elisabeth Kübler-Ross in her lifetime of working with terminally ill patients. Her theory, which was roundly denounced in the late 1960s and early 1970s but has now become a cliché in palliative care circles, postulates that when faced with the diagnosis of a terminal illness, most people go through five stages of reaction. The first is denial, next is anger, then bargaining (listen God, if You get me out of this, I promise to do good deeds for the rest of my life) then depression, then acceptance.

This process is the subject of a superb little film by the National Film Board of Canada called *Why Me?* The five stages are often mentioned in the popular self-help medical literature these days. They even turn up in articles on how to handle losing your job!

In a therapy group I later attended, a woman with lymphoma regaled us with the story of her determined attempts to experience the five stages. We fell about with laughter as Pamela described her astonishment at discovering that not only did you not have to feel each emotion in the order Kübler-Ross had set out, but that it was even OK to skip one. It was a great relief to her to understand that it was normal to bounce back and forth among the stages.

Her account was funny, but it was a sobering moment to recognize how tightly we grasped at theories; we were searching for lifelines and finding them everywhere until they frayed and broke, casting us back into the swim to seek another. We were so obedient in our search, so frenzied that we grasped utterly nonsensical theories, or distorted sensible ones in our earnest desperation to climb out of the sea of cancer.

But early in this journey, I knew no theories, good or bad, no tricks on how to handle the fear. I only knew that self-pity crippled. And anger offered a kind of protection.

Home from the hospital only a few days after surgery, I saw the last half–hour of a TV movie called *Leap of Faith*, about this utterly beautiful young woman who had an incurable lymphoma. At the time I thought it was what I had — a cancer that had spread to the lymph nodes, but in fact lymphomas are tumours that originate in the lymph system. One specific lymphoma is called Hodgkin's disease; all the others are grouped as non-Hodgkin's lymphomas. This exquisite creature tried to meditate her tumour away, and visualize it away, and she'd go to the doctor with her equally beautiful husband, and lie on the examination table with towels artfully draped over her flawless flat-stomached body.

There she was with all her own thick luxurious hair and eyebrows and eyelashes, and her liquid eyes and soft voice and I hated her. She finds a Chinese healer who seems to cure her of her disease through acupuncture, poisonous tea and the installation of a septic tank in the rain. (The healer didn't accept money, only gifts. The husband got to dig the hole and drop the tank in, all in the pouring rain, in about five minutes. Right away I knew this film was lying because we had just tried to do the same thing with a septic tank at the chalet, and it bobbed up in the muddy water like a cork in the sea. It took days of slogging to get it anchored and hooked up.)

Anyway, then the woman goes back to her curmudgeon traditional-medicine doctor who is astounded to discover that her tumour has disappeared. Happy ending as the beautiful couple fades into the sunset. My reaction was violent and rude. Sam and Allen, who were watching it with me, looked askance and said nothing.

The point is, this movie was based on a true story. In my fragile state I found the treatment of the whole subject offensive and scary. Not encouraging or even slightly believable, it just infuriated me. Don't patronize, don't lie, you sanctimonious jerks. I snapped off the TV in disgust. Secretly I wanted to be that vibrant young woman who beat all the odds, right there on TV.

The very next night, there was a documentary on breast cancer. (It seemed that suddenly the media were writing, talking and making films on nothing else.) Called *Destined to Live*, it featured a passel of pretty, articulate, successful women, all with breast cancer — for a week, for seven years, for 18 months, for one year — as the sidebar down the side of the screen said, as each woman spoke into the camera. It was so upbeat, so positive. I knew how Dorothy Parker felt when she read *Winnie the Pooh* and finished her review, "Constant Reader thwowed up."

One woman in the film described with admiring wonder her fiancé's reaction to her breast prosthesis: she touched one breast and said, "This is me." She touched the other and said, "This isn't." He apparently cried out, "Do you think it matters?" And I cried out even louder, "YES, YOU BONEHEAD, IT MATTERS." It might not have mattered to him in all his sensitivity and togetherness, but it would matter to her always. I made bitter comments throughout this film too. I was a real treat.

I did like the feisty woman sheriff in the film, so hearty in her affirmation of life after breast cancer, whose words did not hide her fear and bitterness as she snapped out that men would be more understanding if it were their penis that was at stake. I wonder what her reaction would have been to the doctor who later wrote in *The Lancet* that women should consider preventive mastectomies if they are in a high-risk category for breast cancer. He claimed that women think too much about their breasts (and men don't, of course — think too much about women's breasts, that is).

"After all, [breasts] are just glands and fleshy tissue," he said. Here indeed is a sensitive, compassionate doctor. He went on to make things even worse: "If I thought my beard would increase the percentage risk of getting cancer, I would certainly shave it off."

Is this guy for real? Unfortunately he is, and even more unfortunately, he represents a sizeable cadre of physicians who practise medicine with the sensitivity and understanding of gnats.

Another woman in this film glared at the screen in exasperation, "Friends say to you about getting breast cancer, 'Yes, but you know it's not so bad. I mean anyone could go out tomorrow and get hit by a bus.' What they don't understand is, cancer *is* that bus. You've already been hit."

The film was made by three women with breast cancer. It was an affirmation of faith, but in that early stage of my journey all I could think about was all those other women, the dead ones, the ones whose band down the side of the TV screen would have said, "didn't make it." All the dead ones, lying inarticulate and wasted, they needed a spokeswoman in this film. Unequal representation.

My cynicism in response to these films was a protection from the reality of this new world where I had to find a new persona. These feelings were probably just fine, a kind of cathartic stage to acceptance. However, they must have been hard on people close to me. I found it easier to deal with events by wrapping them in black humour. No one else laughed a lot, though. That would come later, when I met other cancer patients, like Pamela, and three other friends in a support group of five, all with lymphoma. Since we were all in the same boat, we could laugh at the most macabre details without fear of shocking each other into wary pity.

–V–

Simon Says, "Take One Giant Step ... FAST"

*I wake and feel the fell of dark, not day.
What hours, O what black hours we have spent
This night!*

       Gerard Manley Hopkins

The first major step on this journey was surgery. I was shortly to discover what most breast cancer patients know, that although you are encouraged to take one step at a time mentally, the physical treatment is often a hop, skip and a jump, with a paucity of time between to think about where each leap is going to land you. Dr. Simon says Jump, you jump. Simon says There are no options, this is the Way. You don't argue. You line up with the rest of the players, all as shell-shocked as you from the still echoing bulletin that cancer has been detected in *your own body*. You wait for Simon to speak. You hang on his/her every word. At the time no one asks about the rules of the game. Everyone — or at least most everyone; I found out later that there were some brave souls who wouldn't play — does what Simon, The All-Powerful Doctor, decrees.

In my case, Simon said Three Giant Steps: surgery, chemotherapy and radiation. I didn't know about the third step until after I had obediently wobbled through the first two; and for radiation, Simon even gave me a choice. Some choice.

In fact, everyone has choices at every step. At any time you are free to tell Simon to get stuffed. In some cases, that is a wise and brave action, often taken by those whom Bernie Siegel calls "Exceptional Patients." When Simon says, "Die" — or "You have two months to live," which amounts to the same thing — these are the people who say, "Uh uh. I doooon't think so."

Some people, in the terminal stages of cancer, might reject Simon's instructions in a desperate and ill-considered decision to go for the magic cure — extract of the green-lipped Florida wart toad or perhaps a rare and expensive melange of herbs and mushrooms only grown in one secret valley on the north slopes of the Himalayas. Still others turn from Simon in fear, in anger or in resignation that a diagnosis of cancer means instant and painful death, no matter what.

The three stages of medical treatment for breast cancer are commonly referred to by those on the receiving end as "Cut, Poison and Burn." It is a geographic roulette for the patient: if you live in Europe, your doctors might advise quite a different regimen than would a Canadian or North American doctor. In fact, there is emerging from Toronto an approach to the radiation step that differs from the mainstream in the rest of Canada, a branch water that was to sweep me up later.

The variety of treatment protocols is raised in the 1992 report of the Parliamentary Sub-committee on breast cancer. The Committee received contradictory evidence regarding the need to standardize treatment for breast cancer. The submissions from breast cancer sufferers were unanimous, though, about the worry and fear that conflicting treatment *advice* caused. Pat Kelly, the founder of the Burlington breast cancer action group, described the frustration of these women: "Frequently they are told by one oncologist that their approach might be chemotherapy prior to surgery with a subsequent investigation of the need for adjuvant therapy or radiation. In consulting a surgeon, they will be told immediately, we will do surgery and there may or may not be radiation and there may or may not be chemotherapy. There is no systematic approach ... It is most necessary." (*Breast Cancer: Unanswered Questions*, p. 34)

There were equally strong arguments against. "If we have national standards, a prescription laid down by a legislating body, we would end up with a group of physicians who work by a cookbook method, who abrogate thinking and clinical innovativeness to a prescribed protocol. Nothing could be worse ..." (p. 35)

The Committee recommended the middle ground: "We would like to be assured, as would all women in this country, that a diagnosis of breast cancer, whether it be in Newfoundland or Manitoba, would receive treatment that is appropriate, up to date, and relevant for the specific diagnosis and for the patient." (p. 35)

Me too. I'd like to be assured too ... but it is unsettling when you constantly hear of other treatments, other drugs, for the same type and stage of cancer as yours. You wonder always which one is right. There is no absolute "right" one. The most important point in the discussion is the Committee's plea for treatment that is appropriate to the individual patient. Which brings us to the crux of so many of the problems of our present system in which doctors don't see a person but a disease. So question, argue, second guess. Then you become a person because a disease doesn't do any of those things. You might not be the most popular person, but hey, recovering from cancer is not a popularity contest.

My journey began with the "cut" part, perhaps because I had been sent to a surgeon first. Who knows? At the time I did not question the need for surgery, nor do I now. Later stages of treatment did bring the doubt, when I encountered the conflicting rivers of opinion on radiation and the cracked deserts of chemotherapy. In the early days though, I played Simon Says without a murmur.

There was another game called "Let's Pretend." In the lingo, this is called "denial." For me it was survival. To have poured out to the world then that I had breast cancer and that I was having immediate surgery followed by God knows what would have been too heavy a load to carry. When people asked me how I was during those early secret days, mostly I answered brightly, "Fine," and ran for the nearest exit, either figuratively or literally. Family activities all that week led up to my nephew's nuptials, and I didn't want to be the spectre at the wedding.

From later reading about stress and denial and sending your body "live" (rhymes with "sieve" not "dive") messages instead of "die, body, die" ones, I have learned that I had an Attitude problem.

In *Peace, Love and Healing*, Bernie Siegel says, "When someone asks you how you are and you say 'Fine' even though you feel terrible, that's internalizing ... The message you give [your body] when you put on a performance is that you don't want to recover, and the result is that your body cooperates by helping you to die." (p. 33) With his customary gravity, Woody Allen captures the essence of this theory in two lines: "I can't express anger. I internalize it and grow a tumor instead."

However, putting on a performance that week was what got me through it. I would hear myself saying, "I'm fine thanks, how are you?" to friends and half believe it. I am very impressionable. I couldn't have withstood the burden of the worry and fear of those close to me, on top of Allen's and my own. In fact, when I told my brother, Mobe, the night before I was to go into hospital, it wasn't by chance that I chose to speak to him in the dark, standing by the car ready to leave the wedding reception. That way I didn't have to see my own fear mirrored in his eyes. Other people's concern unhinged me.

Of course this approach can be taken to dangerous extremes. Pamela did not tell her parents for almost a year that she had lymphoma. This was indeed a performance, since she lived only a few blocks from them and was undergoing hospital-administered chemotherapy one weekend out of four for months.

Her father told her how much he liked her new hairdo, the first time she wore a wig to hide her sudden baldness. He wondered why she hadn't got it cut like that before. The irony alone of his response must have tempted her to tell all. When finally she did, her parents' hurt was from being excluded from the truth for so long. And her hurt was from the stress of trying to keep up appearances when all her energy was needed for fighting her disease.

Simon Says, "Take One Giant Step ... FAST"

⚭

The day after my nephew's wedding I had to check into the hospital. By one p.m. That way, I got to sit around all afternoon and evening waiting. The nurses insisted that I change into a nightgown immediately, perhaps in case I forgot I was a patient and tried to go home. Matt and Sam came in with flowers and jokes; I felt like an impostor, sitting cross-legged on the bed, feeling physically fine.

That morning, Allen had chopped wood and chopped wood and chopped wood, blistering his hands and dulling his mind with the monotony of the axe splitting into the logs. I prowled around the garden bidding a dramatic farewell to all my plants — those that had survived my special gardening technique of plant and abandon. I had my first inkling that day of a shift in me when I told our neighbours, with no apology, that we would not be contributing to the cost of the fence they were proposing to put up between our back yards, a fence that, according to their plans, would rival the Berlin Wall in its heyday.

"Your fence is pretty low on our priority list," I said, "since a) we don't even want a fence, and b) we have two kids to put through college." *Pardon?* The logic of my first reason was sturdy enough, the logic of the second marginally out of whack.

Before setting out on this journey, I would have compromised or caved in entirely, to keep the peace, to be nice. From somewhere a little steel had entered my soul. Allen had a sudden attack of deafness and kept chopping.

In hospital, a resident visited me with release forms for my signature. The papers said that I was giving permission for the surgeon to perform a mastectomy.

"Oh, no," I said, smiling politely at the mistake. "I am not having a mastectomy. Just a little lump is being taken out."

"And perhaps a bit of tissue around it," I added, wanting to be completely honest. "That is what the doctor said. Look, he even drew me a picture." I hauled out a crumpled bit of paper with Mr. Hulot's diagram on it, a piece of cartography that had helped me stay sane that week, promising as it did that I would not be losing the whole breast. The resident rolled her eyes as if to say, "That's what they all say."

"Before any surgery, the patient must sign these release forms. Now if you could just sign here and here," she said tiredly, indicating the places on the sheet on her clipboard, as if I hadn't spoken.

"I am not having a full mastectomy," I shouted, suddenly losing it. "The surgeon promised."

"This is only a formality, Mrs. Williams," the resident snapped. I was wasting her time, obviously. "Mastectomy can mean anything from the removal of a lump to a radical."

What she really was saying was, "Don't get picky about the details." But dammit, they were my details, and I was rather attached to them.

"Radical what?" I asked very quietly. Allen was with me, and I saw him preparing to intervene; he was a quick learner and was already adept at recognizing the storm signals in my new weather system.

"Radical mastectomy," the resident said, coming full circle, as if that explained everything. Surely she had had this conversation before with other patients, but she apparently was oblivious to the havoc she was causing.

"Mrs. Williams, your surgery cannot be performed if you don't sign these papers."

"So, then I guess it won't be performed." I sat back with folded arms, a belligerent chin and sulky bravado. For the exhausted resident, probably at the end of a 36-hour shift, I was just another task she had to complete late on a Sunday evening before she could leave; get all the pre-op patients to sign their lives away. On these forms the term "mastectomy" was used to refer to any kind of surgery to the breast. She did not explain that. She just grew testy and said that she would have to report my lack of co-operation to the surgeon.

Within the hour, the surgeon sent an emissary to reassure and explain and undo the damage created by the lethal combination of overwork and bureaucracy.

My experience was nothing compared to that of my roommate, a very frightened woman who was told by *her* resident that same evening that the operation she was to have was often unsuccessful and in many cases made the situation even worse. He also told her that she was liable to choke while under anaesthetic and that a tube would be put down her throat to try and prevent this happening. This to a woman whose previous stomach and throat surgery ensured that any tube into that area would probably cause suffocation.

He left her paralysed with fear and, wielding his bedside manner like a bludgeon, proceeded along the hall to reassure his next victim, a fiery young woman who burst into our room to announce her departure from the hospital that instant. She was off to register a formal complaint against this medical miscreant.

The ensuing fuss helped to pass the time: surgeons came in to put out fires; a hospital administrator arrived to take down formal complaints; the whole floor buzzed with excitement.

My surgeon later told me that he spends much of his time undoing the damage caused by well-meaning and not so well-meaning residents. Medical schools are only beginning to teach the importance of reassurance and empathy, and to take seriously the dangers of emotional stress to the patient. The almost exclusive preoccupation with physical treatment emphasizes once again the role of the patient *as* a disease rather than an individual *with* a disease.

It is a sad comment that in the spring of 1992 it was treated as a national news item — an enormous and innovative breakthrough— that a hospital in St. Boniface was introducing the "one-stop shopping" concept to cancer treatment. The hospital now groups appointments so that a newly diagnosed cancer patient can see an oncologist, surgeon, radiologist, the internist, whomever — all at the same time. The old regime, and the one common to most clinics, booked these appointments weeks apart with hours of travel attached to each one. The grouping concept is a great idea — however, it is certainly not new. Cancer patients have been pleading for such a system for 30 years.

That Other Place

As well as living practically on the doorstep of the cancer clinic, I have also been blessed mostly — not always — with caring, humane doctors. I can only surmise, based on the myriad horror stories of others, that I have been very lucky indeed. The surgeon placed me first on the roster early on the morning of surgery to reduce the stressful wait. He spoke to Allen immediately following the operation, visited me in the recovery room and again later in the day back in my room, where I was still seeing two of everybody. Both blurry Mr. Hulots assured me that they had "got it all."

After four days, I went home, trailing a drain from one of the incisions, sore, depressed and no longer numb to what was happening to me. I had lost control of my life — why else would I be lying in bed in a darkened room on a September afternoon wondering if I would make it to Christmas. After having a sort of bath, wearing a plastic grocery bag to keep the bandages dry, I fell — carefully — back into bed. I was worn out by tottering about as if my hips were locked, clutching my right arm across my stomach to prevent it from falling off.

Below the bedroom window, Matt and Sam were playing basketball in the snappy autumn sunlight. They laughed and shouted as the ball thumped off the wall, then one said in a whisper loud enough to raise the crows out of the maple tree across the road, "Shut up, you Binky, Mum's sleeping." And something cracked inside me. Oh God, I did not want to leave them. I did not want to leave Allen, my family, my friends, my life. I did not want to leave my boys with a memory of an invalid mother, closeted in a darkened room.

That day was the beginning of a resolve, a huge resolve that I would do none of those things yet.

-VI-
Just How Fatal Is It?

Basically, all cancer is genetic ... It's not all hereditary, but it's all genetic. What that means is, it's all a gene that screws up.

Susan Ferraro
"You Can't Look Away Anymore"

By the end of that week, there were still no results of the biopsy of the lymph nodes. Such was my state, I didn't want the telephone to ring. Limbo was beginning to look good, a place I could learn to love. Except that I would have gone nuts after about five more minutes of it. Waiting, waiting. For what? Another kick in the teeth. Any residual optimism had drained away with the revolting run-off that filled the shunt still hanging from my side.

Saturday passed in the quiet desperation of time that would not move. Everyone was out — Allen was up at Grand Lake throwing all his energy into the physical building of our dream; Sam was at an art exhibit in town which he was to report on for a school assignment; Matt was at his Saturday job. And I was at home trying to figure out what to do with myself.

I had yet another bath, always my first line of comfort. They were mounting to about nine a day. I slept; I made "greasy" soup just the way Mum used to make it. You clean the refrigerator into a pot, add marrow bones, whatever vegetables are in the house or garden, herbs and water, then simmer for hours. Sometimes it's wonderful. Sometimes it tastes as if you cleaned the refrigerator into a pot ...

I did that. I fed the dogs, the cat and Snicker, the eating machine — Sam's guinea pig. I walked around the house, checking the garden, the size of the zucchini I had planted in the front of the house for decoration. They had turned into monsters because no one had picked them, lurking under the leaves like whales beneath the waves. Checking to make sure the neighbours weren't around, I said hello to the plants I had bid farewell a week earlier, and felt stupid.

No book could hold my attention, the TV was just colour and meaningless voices. I couldn't make any sense of the words. And I waited for Monday. Surely the tests would be done by then.

"Only two have been affected," the surgeon said, when finally the phone call came. "Only two." His voice was apologetic, as if it were his fault that I hadn't a clean slate.

At the time I clung to "only," not understanding the significance of "affected nodes."

The message started to get through when I told my niece the results. Her sharp intake of breath on the phone was a clue that this was indeed not good news. This is my niece the doctor who, through the next few months was a fount of good straight medical information, something I was to find hard to come by.

Most of the doctors and nurses at the cancer clinic I guess assume that patients either don't want to know the medical facts (not statistics and prognosis of survival, but the actual physical medical facts of cancer and treatment) or can't handle them. I would dig and dig for information at every appointment, take it home, mull over it, worry it, study it and get my niece to fill in the huge gaps left through either the doctors' hedging or my wrong questions.

I learned very quickly that, according to statistics, any affected nodes lessen the chance of long-term survival considerably because it means that the disease has metastasized — it's already on its way to other parts of the body.

Breast cancer is staged according to size of tumour, the number of lymph nodes involved, whether it has spread to the chest wall or other organs. The following is from PDQ, a computer on-line data base of information on cancer treatment, maintained by the National Cancer Institute in the U.S. PDQ is continually updated, or to quote from the introduction, "reviewed each month by cancer experts." The library at the Ontario Cancer Clinic, Ottawa Civic Hospital, and probably most medical libraries throughout the country, will do a search at minimal or no cost.

Stages of breast cancer
Once breast cancer has been found (diagnosed), more tests will be done to find out if the cancer has spread from the breast to other parts of the body (staging). The doctor needs to know the stage to plan treatment. The following stages are used for breast cancer:

Stage O Breast cancer in situ
This is very early breast cancer (sometimes it is called noninvasive carcinoma). Cancer is only found in a local area and in only a few layers of cells. Other terms for this type of breast cancer are intraductal carcinoma or ductal carcinoma in situ and lobular carcinoma in situ.

Stage I
The cancer is no bigger than 2 centimetres (cm) — about 1 inch — and has not spread outside the breast.

Stage II
The cancer is from 2 to 5 cm — from 1 to 2 inches — and/or has spread to the lymph nodes under the arm (axillary nodes).

Stage III
The cancer is bigger than 5 cm — about 2 inches — and has spread to the tissues near the breast (chest wall); or the cancer is smaller than 5 cm but has spread to many of the lymph nodes under the arm; or the cancer has spread to lymph nodes near the collarbone.

Stage IV
The cancer has spread to other organs of the body, most often the bones, lungs, liver, or brain.

Inflammatory breast cancer
Inflammatory breast cancer is a special class of breast cancer that is rare. The breast looks as if it is inflamed because of its red appearance and warmth. The skin may show signs of ridges and wheals or it may have a pitted appearance. It tends to spread quickly.

Recurrent
Cancer has come back (recurred) after previous treatment.

At stage O, the National Cancer Institute gives the five-year survival rate as 95 percent. At stage II (where those two infected nodes put me) the five-year survival is 66 percent.

Those are scary numbers. At the time, I must have read or been told these statistics since they are noted in my journal, but I forgot them fast. And I keep forgetting them in my search to find better odds, because if you look hard enough you are bound to find them.

-VII-
The Search for Better Odds

*Treating cancer is a matter of statistics —
we go with the numbers.*

Oncologist quoted in Chopra, *Quantum Healing*

Reading a lot about cancer is a powerful exercise for an eclectic mind — you gather a fact here, a fact there, put them all together and what have you got? A passel of conflicting facts.

Each book or article gives you a definitive — and different — set of statistics and expectations, serving them up with such certainty. Depending on their circumstances, readers cling to these little lifeboats of percentages in the sea of conflicting research and opinion. But statistics are highly suspect, ready to sink leaving bubbles of misinformation to confound the searchers even more.

For example, examine closely the statistical analysis of the likelihood of developing breast cancer if someone in your family already has or had it. If your sister has breast cancer, you have a 75 percent chance of getting it too. If your mother had breast cancer, you have a 50 percent chance of getting it. Taken to their logical conclusion, odds are that if your mother, sister, grandmother and aunt all have the disease, you have a statistical likelihood of 150 percent of getting breast cancer. In other words you haven't got a snowball's chance. I love putting this spin on statistics. It helps maintain an equilibrium, as does the loony claim quoted in a Canadian research journal on corrections that "recent figures indicate that 43% of all statistics are utterly worthless." The author of that article goes on to put statistics in their place: "A statistic is just a number which, if calculated correctly, tells us something about a group of numbers." (*Forum*, 5.3)

Another instance of conflicting, confusing, confounding information with which the air waves are loud: women with breast cancer are not officially "declared cured" for 16 years after the occurrence.(Fine); five years after the occurrence (conversation with oncologist, Ontario Regional Cancer Clinic); eight years (conversation with surgeon, Ottawa Civic Hospital); three years (Chopra) and 20 years (*Breast Cancer: Unanswered Questions*).

Once again, statistics are to blame for these moving targets. Such time frames are simply for the purposes of statistical analysis. They may offer some solace or goal for us patients, but they are also false. You make it to the end of five or eight or 16 years and shout "Hurray, I am cured." And the next day you find a lump in the remaining breast, or develop symptoms that indicate a growth in your liver. Is it comforting to believe that these are new cancers rather than a development of the old one?

Well, perhaps. If it is a new one, you have another chance at recovering (if it is breast cancer), because the odds against you beating a recurrence of the same breast cancer are low, low, low. At least that's what my oncologist said. PDQ Cancer information data base says that too, only more gently: "Breast cancer that comes back (recurs) can often be treated, but usually cannot be cured." Yet in the last five years I have met many, many women with a recurrence of breast cancer who have long outlived the 14-month average survival after the second bout. One incredibly gutsy young woman had eight recurrences in as many years. Each time she just picked herself up off the canvas and came back punching. For eight years, she fought with everything she had — traditional treatment, alternative treatment, an amazing spirit, humour, bravery — until the final bout.

I think of her often, her gusts of laughter as she related an anecdote, her anger at her disease, her courage in the face of the pain and nausea of treatment and her powerful, engulfing will to live.

ളൟ

After the first shock of diagnosis and surgery began to wear off, I wanted the facts; I wanted certainties; I wanted someone to tell me the truth about it all, a truth that wouldn't shift and waver with everything I read. At least, that's what I thought I wanted. Really I was searching for someone who would tell me for certain sure that there was a route out of this country.

It was an impossible quest. The only truth I found was that there isn't any. At least no absolute truth, just versions and layers like Durrell's *Alexandria Quartet*. Each person's cancer is his or her own truth.

Cancer will not behave in a predictable fashion. There are averages and statistics, but that's it. "Cell division is a carefully considered and well-thought-out decision — except in the case of cancer. Cancer is wild, anti-social behaviour, whereby a single cell reproduces itself without check, heeding no signals from anywhere except, apparently, its own demented DNA. Why this occurs, no one knows." (Chopra, p. 46)

There are more than 200 different cancers, for most of which there is no known cause or cure. That about sums it up. *Everyone's Guide to Cancer Therapy* wistfully states that, "In fact, cancer remains something of a mystery." (Dollinger *et al*, p.3) And this is in a *guide* to cancer! It is actually a very good textbook approach to cancer therapy, thorough, honest and well-written. Its section on breast cancer is complete, easy to follow — and depressing. But it does provide the clarity of the few facts available, and does not wander off into averages and statistics which are OK in theoretical discussions, as distant information about something that is not actually eating away inside *you*. Direct application of such tools designed to bring order and understanding to a disease, the reality of which lies in its very lack of order, does not often bring comfort. Although I suppose if I were in the 95 percent long-term survival range I would take greater comfort in the numbers game.

Risk factors, like survival rates, are another area of conflicting information. What causes breast cancer to strike one woman and not the next? Again, depending on the book you read, the documentary you watch, the doctor you listen to, these factors range from too much repressed emotion to not enough carrots. The most common (not in order) are:

- early menstruation and late menopause
- history of breast cancer in the family
- low fertility
- use of oral contraceptives over a long period
- alcohol consumption
- caffeine consumption (although Dollinger *et al*, p. 243, says this is *not* a risk. Yay.)
- fat consumption
- food additives
- body shape
- environmental toxins
- radiation (including too many mammograms)
- hormone replacement therapy
- stress
- having had cancer before

The biggest risk of all is just being a woman, according to *Breast Cancer: Unanswered Questions*, because in 60 to 70 percent of women with breast cancer, none of the other risk factors is present. And that one is a difficult one to avoid, at least once you are born. The final answer is that no one really knows where or why cancer strikes. The one positive aspect of this lottery is that you can't blame yourself when you win ... lose.

Another area of confusion: success rates of treatment. Some studies suggest that treatment of breast cancer is more successful than it was 10 years ago. Others state that although the percentage of breast cancer survivors is the same as 10 years ago, really the treatment is more successful because there are more people with breast cancer these days. This kind of analysis makes me crazy. Are we talking good news or bad news here? Hard to say.

The predominant claim is that the long-term survival rate among women with breast cancer is not keeping pace with the relentless increase of incidence of the disease. And this is not just in Canada. Recent data indicate a 55 percent increase in Japan, 10 percent in Sweden and former West Germany, and 16 percent in Brazil. (*Breast Cancer: Unanswered Questions,* p. 4)

When you have breast cancer you don't want to have to weigh all the information. You yearn for better statistics even though a lot of the time you claim not to believe them anyway. After all, they are just numbers, right? And we all know how numbers can be manipulated to come up with the desired result, whether for political, financial, medical, ethical or just plain perverse reasons. Unfortunately, right now there are no better statistics, no firmer facts about breast cancer. Even *Everyone's Guide to Cancer Therapy* chooses its words carefully: it doesn't make any claims for higher success rates of treatment, for example; what it does say (p. 241) is, "Over the past twenty years, the approach to evaluating and treating breast cancer has changed considerably."

So be prepared to spend a lot of waking hours in a revolving door. Where you shoot out is pure roulette ... but usually right where the popular press is waiting to propel you back in again. I have found, in print, theories and opinions to back up every single shibboleth of cancer. It is a jungle of misconstrued, misinformed, shallow, badly researched, skewed reporting.

Two days after the beginning of my fifth chemo treatment I read that, "Catching cancer before it can spread through the human body almost always means the difference between life and death. Medical experts say that nearly all cancer patients whose disease has begun to spread at the time of detection have little chance of survival." When you casually scan such an article, you might think, "Uh huh, makes sense." But it doesn't. Such a generalized summary flagrantly disregards staging of the disease and individual circumstances. The bone of "nearly" tossed in as a qualifier is not enough for this terrier.

Those of us motivated by our very own cancer speeding away from the original tumour site read such statements with pain, then with care and then with fury. We actually parse the sentences and dig out the meaning as a way of protecting ourselves from the anguish of carelessly chosen, ill-informed words.

"The difference between life and death" means falling off a 500-foot cliff onto sharp rocks. Or not. If you've got metastatic cancer, you don't necessarily keel over dead the minute you find out; rather, you are freighted with the knowledge that you have a statistically lower chance of living a naturally long life.

And "little chance of survival": does this mean that you might not make it to the consulting room door? Or that you won't live forever, as will all the other people in the world who don't have cancer? No, it means that you are more likely to die sooner than later. Statistically. It is essential to remember that all this talk is based on statistics, a necessary foundation from which to direct research, but lethal in the hazy texts of superficial reporting.

I read this article with a mind clouded by chemotherapy and depression deepened by the cheap coin of a catchy lead of a reporter facing a deadline. Why then was I going through chemo, why did I have surgery, if the odds were so stacked against me? What do you believe in all you read and hear?

Very early in this journey, I elected, in order to stay sane, to be selective and biased and totally tunnel-visioned in seeing only the encouraging and positive. However, that first year after diagnosis, an occasional line of print still slithered through a chink in the armour and like a switchblade carved a hole in my consciousness, large enough for the thought to take root: maybe I won't even make it to the first hurdle.

My defences were stronger than I realized. In the midst of chemotherapy, I read an article by an American journalist who had breast cancer and whose journey was identical to mine, the same surgical procedure, chemo treatments and radiation, right down to her surgeon telling her too that the lump was "99 percent certain" to be benign. An identical journey except for one thing — her cancer had not metastasized — the lymph nodes were clear.

Her bleak angry account did not depress me. In fact I was heartened by reading about a case so similar and, I shudder to think of this now, I even felt smug, because here was this woman with less cancer than me, and she was whining about it. Not me. I wasn't whining and lashing out. I was just a Goody Two Shoes, a Bad Thing for the immune system so the self-help literature says. I still think this was one case when self-delusion was a Good Thing, a protective crouch against being mugged by reality.

I read this article again a year after my last radiation treatment. This time it depressed the hell out of me, not because of its mournful tone but because of the total honesty and accuracy of her account. She ends on an upbeat note, but it sounds forced; her spirit is bruised and still cowering from the whole experience.

"My trust in the future is no longer seamless," she writes. "I still feel it's possible for my life to shatter again. In an instant, I could be incarcerated by illness, deprived of momentum, of the ongoing enterprise that is my life."(Bergholz) Her words sum up one of the certain legacies of breast cancer: the tangible proof of the frailty of life, the ever-present nudge of mortality.

-VIII-
Wrestling with Reality

Until death, it is all life.
Cervantes, *Don Quixote*

Waiting. Waiting for calls from the clinic, the surgeon, the oncologist, the X-ray department, the nuclear medicine crowd. I was now measuring out my life not in coffee spoons, but in test results. First was the biopsy of the lymph nodes, 11 of which had been scooped out from inside my shoulder, like seeds from a pomegranate; then ultrasound, bone scan, X-rays and blood tests. Later it would be the iron grip of treatment and after that, the two-month check-ups, then three-month, each one bringing its own battery of tests and examinations, its own measure of stress with the regular refocusing on the spectre of recurrence.

This was not *Waiting for Godot* stuff, because for Beckett, waiting is the human condition, it is the way we all live, all the time; no, this was the specific, mind-arresting wait for news that could immediately alter the course of my life. It was the out-of-control, news-from-another-planet stuff of nightmares.

Immediately after the operation and confirmation of metastatic cancer in the lymph nodes I was sent for a bone scan and an ultrasound examination. These were to establish "base study data" before the next stage of treatment. Neither of these tests can detect microscopic disease, but they do pinpoint any developed cancer sites. The oncologist assured me that she was 99 percent certain that the tests would not find any cancer, a phrase that now sent fear scudding through me. Given its previous record in my life, it did not reassure.

The ultrasound is no big deal. In fact, it was a nice break since the only part of it that could remotely be called uncomfortable was the lubricating ointment they smear on your body to allow the scan to slide easily. It was freezing. My insides looked like a lunar landscape until the technician flicked on the colour. Then I looked like a weather map of the Great Lakes system.

The bone scan was equally painless. It is a disturbing notion, though, to know that you are being injected on purpose with a radioactive dye which courses through your body like pollution in a stream. After a two-hour wait to ensure full saturation, I lay about two inches beneath an enormous grinding machine that for the next hour clunked down my body inch by inch like a manual typewriter. The dye highlights "hotspots" on a screen, confirming the absence or presence of cancer cells.

Both tests were negative. By then I fully expected to light up like a "Christmas tree in July," the shocking description of the bone scan results of the protagonist in *Sailing*, Susan Kenney's fine, tough novel about cancer. So tough that I banged it shut at that very point, too late to prevent the cancer Christmas tree image to brand my already embattled brain. This was not escapist literature. What was I doing reading such books? This was the reality of fiction underscoring the reality of my own life; I was really sick of reality.

When you are first told that you have cancer the reality doesn't stick right away. It does indeed sink in, to a degree — like a very sharp axe square between the eyes, splitting you into two people. One of you gibbers with fear, the other copes. And it's only later that you find out that the coping side is what might have got you into trouble in the first place.

In the hospital the night before surgery, I wrote "Tomorrow morning early, instead of diving into the work day, I will be operated on for breast cancer. That word — cancer — still after six days I do not associate with me. It is what other people

That Other Place

have ... The fear comes in waves and literally curdles my stomach. But then there are stretches when it is dulled and I feel OK and busy and normal." This was to be the pattern for the next two years, and probably will be the pattern forever in varying degrees. Because for cancer, we read "death." The varying degrees depend on the time of night, the latest news, the last book you have read.

It is not only the person newly diagnosed as having cancer who has a shaky grasp on the reality of the disease. Friends and relations also struggle with denial, holding with tenacity the assumption that cancer is what you read about in those weepy articles in women's magazines. Partly it is the brain's way of cushioning the blow, but occasionally the cushioned blow rebounds back in a rabbit punch that truly knocks the wind out of you.

Shortly after I had been pole-axed into this new country, and was lying whimpering across the border from my old life, a very close friend, Andy, and I were talking about how breast cancer seemed to be on the increase, at least in our lives. Mr. Hulot had told me that he was now diagnosing, on average, three breast cancers a week — this was one practice, of one surgeon, in one hospital, in one medium-sized city. Feed that fact into the statistics hopper and what emerges is a lot of breast cancer. This, coupled with the willingness of more and more people to talk about their disease, has cancer in almost every headline.

Once it was that cancer, along with alcoholism, was a shameful affliction. Now it seems everyone has it and says so. The medical scuttlebutt is that everyone will die of cancer if they live long enough. That's the kind of statement that keeps logicians awake at night, but the kind that slides trippingly off the tongue in the middle of a freewheeling discussion unfettered by mere fact.

Andy said, fearfully, "Breast cancer is everywhere. It could happen to any of us."

I looked at her in astonishment. It *had* happened to any of us. Me. For her, my reality hadn't taken hold. She was back in that other country, forgetting that I had already crossed the border.

Wrestling with Reality

Shaken and feeling more alone than ever, I drifted in a kind of ether of denial and acceptance at the same time. Just where was I? Which world?

The answer, for the first little while, was both. I swung back and forth between my old life with the old priorities trying to cling to their positions, and the new ones, which knocked the old worry-list galley west. These were not the anxieties that move mistily through everyone's lives, but the looming solidity of a huge liner gliding out of the fog, taking on substance and intent as it bears down on you.

After surgery, despite the Simon Says Game, I felt that I had choices. I had had choices before surgery too, but everything happened so fast, and I was so derailed by the diagnosis and the total certainty of the surgeon's advice, I did not question what had to be the next step. I do not question it now in retrospect, but I can understand that in some instances people do question and reject surgery. Choices are their right and do not belong only to the Simons.

Within the stress and fear of suddenly coming face-to-face with your own mortality, thoughtful decisions do not come easy. What came easy for me was to do exactly what I was told. Like a robot computerized to respond to voice commands. Go to the hospital on Sunday. OK. Wait until Monday. OK. Be operated on. OK. Beyond that I shorted out.

Now I had to make decisions. Simon said, chemotherapy. I never argued with that. But what kind? Would I go into a clinical study which randomly selected one of three arms of treatment using different combinations of drugs and radiation? Or would I go to another clinic for a second opinion as Sylvia, my forerunner on this course, had done just a few months earlier? It was her response to Simon saying, CHEMOTHERAPY. In spades.

"Absolutely not," she had said flatly. "I will not take chemotherapy. I am not good at being a sick person." And she took her records to another hospital in another city — to another game where the Simons put her on a very mild regimen of drugs. She urged me to do the same thing — go to a bigger centre, get a second opinion.

That Other Place

A lot of the books tell you to do that too. So pretty soon the guilt kicked in because I didn't *want* a second opinion. One was enough. All my instincts said, do what has to be done, here in Ottawa. The initial treatment for my stage and kind of cancer would be the same wherever I went, or so I thought. It turns out that it could have differed fairly dramatically— a full mastectomy instead of a lumpectomy, radiation first, then chemo; no radiation; or no chemo. But these were choices I did not know were out there. At the time, judging from Sylvia's experience, I felt that whatever treatment I needed — which of course was carved in the clever stone of research and the all-knowing experience of the Simons — might be offered to me in kinder language, it might be adapted because of my mental attitude — but nothing would change the fact that I had cancer that had to be dealt with fast and hard. So Sylvia's route was not the one for me.

Everybody has their own way to follow. I think the main secret of recovering from, or at least living with, cancer is finding your own way. It must be your choice, you must feel comfortable with your choice. Then you have a jump start on finding the way back.

After surgery and the news that "*only* two lymph nodes are affected ... " I had about three weeks to come to terms with the next step. Before it all began to sink in, I thought, "Oh well, two isn't so bad."

I was partly right. Two wasn't as bad as three, five, 12. The whole ball of wax. My first visit to the oncologist set me right, and set me right back on my ear. Here was a doctor who did not mince words. She clipped them out like tiny bits of shrapnel: "With breast cancer," she said with a directness that crucified, "we only have one kick at the can. In your case, we have a good chance if we attack hard. That means aggressive treatment, because there is no survival of a second bout." Hey, what happened to the gentle euphemisms?

I heard my voice echoing weakly, "No survival?"

"None. But if we catch it now, you have a good chance."

A good chance for what? It appeared she said, "A good

chance to live five more years."

As it turned out that isn't exactly what she said but that is what I heard. I heard a lot of strange things in those early days. Communication wasn't too clear between the old world and my new one. But this "five year" measuring stick was hard to accept, yet another piece of the new landscape of this ferocious country.

In the old days, at least two months before this conversation took place, lifetime was forever. You didn't think in allotted chunks of time, you didn't parcel out the future, you just assumed that it stretched out before you, and only other people died.

Suddenly, the future had atrophied. Five years. And that was the bright side. I could come to the end of the road as soon as I stepped out of the present. That was the beginning of a struggle to rethink a lot of assumptions. Later, when I read Bernie Siegel's book, *Love, Medicine and Miracles*, I discovered that was one of his main messages. "Good morning folks. You are all going to die," he said at the opening of his workshop in Toronto. Or words to that effect. There was a gasp from the audience. I just nodded smugly. I already knew that secret. *Then*, right then, I did. I had a firm grasp on the whole concept, made firmer by the inroads of chemo treatment, the lingering pain of surgery and the echo down the days of the first time the surgeon finally said straight out, "You have breast cancer."

Bernie was just stating the obvious, right? Wrong. For most of us it is the most unobvious thing in our lives. And what's more, society reinforces our ostrich stance by promising everlasting life if we use anti-aging skin cream, drink water, don't drink water, drink red wine, don't drink red wine, stop smoking, jog every day, don't jog every day, ride a bicycle to work, dancercize, exercise, eulogize youth and we will be young forever. None of the ads say use this cream and you won't have wrinkles for five years; take a membership in our health club and you should last about five years longer. They say take a *lifetime* membership in our club. Which encourages us all to forget that a lifetime could be as long as the next minute.

That Other Place

For most of us, it takes some kind of epiphany to grasp this utterly commonplace bit of wisdom. And it takes constant work to keep remembering it, undermined as we are by magazine articles such as: "Breast cancer update: At some time in their lives, one of every ten women will be told by their doctors they have breast cancer. All of them will be shattered by the news; many will eventually die." (Doheny, p. 39)

And the rest? They will live forever, already? We will all "eventually die," dammit, even those fellows in Dallas who claim they have isolated the DNA that controls aging and that it is now within science's grasp to allow us to live for 100,000 years. Yikes. What a concept. But it is downright mean of all these articles to suggest that the only people who die, ever, are those with cancer.

Whoever said, "No one gets out of this life alive" may have been stating the obvious, but most people secretly believe they will do just that; it's everyone else who dies. This form of protective thinking allows you to deny the obvious: that life is terminal too; just as terminal as cancer. It's all a question of degree ... Cancer tends to rip those brain blinkers right off. It is a sobering moment when you come face to face with your own mortality.

Even with cancer coursing through our bodies, most of us circle the reality of our own deaths like a terrier circling a porcupine. The terrier rushes in, snaps and backs off yelping, circles again, darts back in, and out, weaving a little dance, two lunges forward, one lunge back. The eventual mouthful of quills has the same inevitability as death and taxes; but that terrier stalks the porcupine with the same optimism with which most of us look at our own deaths — a stupid misplaced conviction that we will avoid the quills and live forever. Forever, of course, could mean 20 years or even two — it is a chunk of time that is not now, nor ever will be. Our deaths are always in the future, a station at which we will never arrive. What brings that station a little closer up the line for breast cancer victims is a new ache or pain, another article or book that looks on the dark side, or the death of a friend on this same journey.

-IX-
Brief Encounter with the Technocrats

They told me, at the cancer clinic, that I was eligible to be part of a research study in experimental treatment for breast cancer. Eligible. Odd word, suggesting that I had worked hard, behaved myself, followed all the rules, ate the right foods, and Was Chosen. In fact, eligibility depended on more mundane considerations: size of tumour, whether the cancer had spread to the lymph nodes, number of nodes affected, age and general health.

The study concentrated on three different forms of treatment, one to which the patient is randomly assigned by computer. There was the conventional chemotherapy for breast cancer that, supposedly, lasted for six months; there was the conventional treatment with a different combination of drugs; and a third that included longer treatment and a stronger drug.

The oncologist talked about ethics and not being able to break the code when I asked if the treatments they were studying were more effective. They did not know yet. What they were sure of was that the two other treatments were no *less* effective than the conventional one, that the stronger drug definitely caused complete hair loss, more intense nausea and vomiting. This had to be weighed against the possibility of a more certain cure.

OK, I said. I would consider it. *Consider* it. The study was not run by the oncologist, but by a clinician whose name was Bawlotski or Blitski, or maybe Bornwithnoheartski; his forehead bulged with brains and gleamed with the fervour of a dedicated

That Other Place

scientist. He worked with cells and microscopes and tiny sheets of blood-stained glass, forgetting apparently that they came from human beings. I don't think he had seen a real person in 20 years. They might have swum into his ken, like me, but he didn't see them. What he saw were cells and blood in a different shape of test tube.

His hooded, flat, yellow eyes flicked from me to Allen like car headlights shining on a pair of rabbits.

"Here is const firm," he said, handing me a sheaf of papers. Const firm? Either my ears or his English was not working. Was it even English? As he spoke, I occasionally recognized a word — such as "terminal" or "death" — words that strike terror into the bravest of hearts. This man would set hospital public relations back 50 years. His professional manner was one he had apparently learned from books on Nazi Germany. A patient was his or her disease. Period.

Through the spikes of abused English came the occasional message. The study was going to be closed in two days; they had enough subjects; it had been going five years. In Pidsbg. Where? Pidsbg. Pittsburgh. I was beginning to catch on. The "const firm" started with "I have been informed that ..." A consent form! Of course. Four pages long, it consented to torture and death. It had been written by a pack of lawyers all with "libel suit" stamped on their foreheads. It was terrifying.

"Yer hair fall out, yis," Blitski said, his voice rising with excitement.

The consent form required that you agree to radiation therapy. Twenty-two days of it. I had already been told by the oncologist that she would not recommend radiation for me. I told the Beam.

His shoulder twitch suggested I was splitting hairs. What's 22 days of unnecessary radiation in the cause of science.

"Iss not included in study," Blitski said, shifting his stare to the corner of the ceiling. I turned to see if the paint was blistering. Why did I not believe him?

He talked about the study some more, his glare flashing on and off like a lamp with a faulty connection. His eyes gleamed brightest when he was talking about the more unpleasant details.

"Durink surgery, the cancer cells spret," he said happily.

"During?"

"Yiss, yiss, durink."

"You mean, while the operation is going on? Right then?" I asked in disbelief.

"Yiss, yiss. The cells spret to other cuts." He waved his arms in excitement.

Dear God, the visuals were sudden and in technicolour. The knife does its work and out pop the cancer cells all racing for dear life up the breast looking for new hiding places. Sort of like that game we used to play, Run My Ten Sheep Run.

Blitski told me that it would be an honour — for me — to be included in the study; that my participation could help countless others many years down the road. At least I think that's what he said. He did not mince words, he obliterated them.

I asked about other side-effects. His stare slid upwards again. This time a scorched spider fell from the top of the window and lay twitching on the carpet. Struck by lightning, I guess.

Blitski rubbed his hands. "Blot in urn," he said with satisfaction. "Blot in urn?" I repeated dazedly. "What is that?"

Was he leaping over the torture to the death part? Was he saying that after his treatment I would be a mere blot in the funeral urn, a smudge of ash left after being radiated, injected and dosed with such glee? I felt my mind unhook into a surreal landscape of cemeteries of stone chalices, each with small blots inching their way to the top, their little blot arms stretching to the sky.

"Iss red. Iss not good. Blot in urn, you see?"

Absolutely, I did not see. For the third time, and with growing desperation, I whispered, "blot in urn?" Each time Blitski repeated it after me, only louder. Our chorus was interrupted by Allen's low interjection: "Blood in the urine," he spoke quietly so as not to attract the Beam.

In the end, I chose not to go into the study. It was one of the few easy decisions on this journey.

-X-
Simon Says, "Take Another Giant Step: Chemotherapy"

> *Extreme remedies are very appropriate for extreme diseases.*
> Hippocrates: *Aphorism I*

The research study offered me was one of the few easy steps on this route to bypass, mainly because of how it was offered, not because of what it might or might not be able to accomplish. Next main step now was chemotherapy. Chemotherapy. A bogey word that used to float around out there in other people's ether. If I thought about it at all, it was with a slight shudder and a "Thank God, I don't have to have it." Touch wood. I must have touched stone.

The word "chemotherapy" has such an armour of horrible mystery about it that I hadn't even realized that it was simply a treatment of drugs, chemicals. Instead of taking aspirin for a headache, you took chemo for a cancer, a less than subtle method to curb normal cells gone haywire. Its lack of refinement, its scattergun approach that takes out good cells as well as bad, has led to its hit-and-miss reputation. But it is up against a formidable opponent.

Cancer is endowed with a mad genius, while drugs are simple-minded. So the oncologist resorts to a much cruder assault, a form of poisoning. Anti-cancer drugs are generally toxic to the entire body, but because cancer cells are growing

Simon Says, "Take Another Giant Step: Chemotherapy"

at a much faster rate than most normal cells, they ingest more poison and die off first. One hopes. It is a calculated risk. Often it is a race to see which die first, the white blood cells which are essential to a healthy immune system, or the cancer cells which the immune system is trying to fight off with the fast-depleting aid of the white blood cells. It is a fine scenario for a war movie if it only weren't being shot in your own body.

There are many ways to take chemotherapy – there are pills, injections, intravenous, drips, portopacks; there is a relatively new zapping technique in which the drugs are shot straight into the tumour. The intravenous method was my passport to the chemo room in the cancer clinic at the Ottawa Civic Hospital.

That first morning I was scared witless but wearing a brave face. Here was the routine. First, the blood tests; for these you take a number, just like waiting in line at the deli counter in Loblaws. Or you push a buzzer by the blood-room door to summon a nurse. After the first month, this always made me think of Pavlov's dogs; I'd ring the buzzer and immediately my throat would go dry, my veins would start a frenzied twitch away from the needle that wasn't even in sight yet.

Before all of this I never minded having needles, giving blood; none of the trappings of normal medical maintenance ever fazed me. Now, my brain stutters at the thought of such innocent pricks. My pain threshold over these last few years has sunk into a spongy swamp of whimpering and thrashing at the gentlest activities to do with veins or needles. I was never a pretty sight at the dentist, but now dental assistants come in from outer offices just to see how much white of my eyes shows when the dentist tries to put in the freezing.

In the blood room, the nurse extracts blood, sometimes from a finger or a thumb, sometimes from a wrist, the back of the hand or inside the elbow. She fills little vials with your blood and taps them authoritatively with a pen. This is to change it back from the ice water it turned into when she started wielding the needle.

She scrapes little droplets of blood onto glass slides, labelling everything in triplicate; she asks you your name while checking the request form, to make sure you haven't turned into someone else before her very eyes. Which you have, of course. You came to the clinic as a normal functioning human being, perhaps wondering what you were going to do on the weekend, planning a dinner party around carrot juice, but by the time you have been tapped like a maple tree, you are transformed into another personality — someone controlled from outside, without the ability to make decisions, reduced to a disease with a number.

So, as Number 12, you obediently go down the hall, as directed, and wait in the waiting room. And wait. You wait for the results of the blood tests, you wait for a chair or bed in the chemo room, you wait for the chemo nurses to come back from coffee-break, you wait while the entire staff rushes past you in response to a mysterious code 999 over the PA system. You wait while they stroll back. You wait while the entire staff rushes past you at the end of their shift. You wait. Which, in the circumstances, is a lot better than arriving.

You hear your name being called. You wish that you weren't you. You wish that another Ms. Williams would jump to her feet, smiling bravely. No one does, so you do. A nurse with a chart beckons to you from the door of the chemo room.

Your response depends on whether this is your first treatment or whether you have been here before. If it is your first, you are apprehensive. If it is your second treatment, you are apprehensive and slightly sick. It goes downhill from there.

The nurses are friendly, reassuring, understanding. The room wears a disguise of pretty non-institutional bedspreads and bright splashy shawls. These do not mask the sad, grey faces of the people beneath them, nor the network of wires leading to bared arms. Sun streams through the wall of windows. You hate it.

A nurse, your personal one for the duration, checks your chart several times to ensure that she has the right patient and that she is administering the correct drugs, the correct dosages; she checks to see if there is a note on your chart about your previous reactions. Did you throw up, faint, cry, punch out a doctor, snarl at a well-meaning volunteer?

Simon Says, "Take Another Giant Step: Chemotherapy"

You sit in a lazy-boy recliner. It doesn't fool you. It is not lazy, boy, it is definitely not lazy. Or easy.

"Pop this under your tongue," the nurse says, giving you a tiny pill or two, intended to quell the nausea.

The tube is inserted into one of the few veins that has not fled before the probing fingers of the attendant as she looks for a new site for the needle. (It is almost three years after my chemotherapy treatments and as I write, I can feel the nausea building in my throat, the shaky sensation inside my arms and legs, the churning of my stomach.)

The drugs start to pour through your body, an indescribable, invasive, obscene sensation.

For me, each treatment was different, none of them my favourite way to spend the day. But the first one, on a sunny October morning, had very little immediate physical aftereffect. I had gone to the clinic alone and walked home from the hospital in the warm autumn wind, scuffing through the swirling leaves along the sidewalk down Ruskin Avenue, over to Holland and down to Byron, past the tennis courts littered with the detritus of autumn.

The stately old maples in our neighbourhood on Java and Kenora streets were ablaze; opposite our house, the biggest of them all towered above rooftops, a glorious deep bronze, a proud ancient tree that had survived against all odds. That day was one of those delicious gifts of a day that Canada delivers up at the end of summer, a day full of energy and promise, rather than one presaging winter. I sat for a moment on our front steps and looked up at the giant maple and wondered if I would see it in its autumn glory ever again. Not because it was sick, but because I was.

My shoulder, arm and breast ached from the surgery three weeks earlier; my other arm tingled where the tube had been, but I could feel the day lift me out of the reality of my journey. The fear of chemo was worse than the actuality, so I thought, that day. I was so cocky — what was all this talk about feeling so sick after a chemo treatment, this advice to go with someone who could deliver you home safely? In fact, why did the doctor

That Other Place

say you mustn't drive a car after a treatment? Look at me, walking a mile, slowly and a little tottery, but nevertheless walking. I wasn't going to let this stuff get *me* down. I was made of stronger mettle.

Hubris is not restricted to arrogant Greeks who thought they could control their own fates.

Once a week for two weeks out of each month, I had chemotherapy by intravenous; during those same two weeks I took a clutch of pills every morning, accompanied by an anti-nausea drug called Stemital®, which I consumed like candy in the last few weeks of treatment. In those early days, I thought I was only supposed to take it each morning. And so obedient was I, that even though the nausea built up during the day from the whack of chemo pills each morning, I dared not take any more. Finally it dawned on me that it was my body, and I could tell better than anyone else what helped and what was useless in the face of the nausea.

My experience with chemo is not typical, because no one's is. Everyone's reaction is individual; bodies, attitudes, drugs and dosages vary; methods of delivery are different. But most important, there seems to have been some genuine breakthrough in both the accuracy of administering the drugs and in the pain and nausea medications that accompany chemo. Ask about them. Demand them. Be a total pain in the neck to the medical profession if you start getting the runaround. Ask about marijuana, now being prescribed as an aid to dealing with pain and nausea. A friend who had lymphoma sailed through two weeks of a concentrated, daily regimen of treatment on the wings of the drug. There is no doubt the quality of her life was improved dramatically by the small dose of Mexican gold, or whatever it was, so frowned upon by many. It strikes me that the immorality of this issue would be if such treatment was denied rather than administered to a patient who requested it. My friend, aided by her family, had to fight hard for the marijuana, using up what little energy she had in the frustration and anger of dealing with the medical bureaucracy, energy she could have used to fight her disease.

Simon Says, "Take Another Giant Step: Chemotherapy"

The point is this: it is *your* body, *your* pain, *your* life. Your very first responsibility is to yourself — do whatever it takes.

⚭

Chemotherapy is like a crab. Its two big pincers are hair loss and nausea. Most breeds have a lot of extra pincers as well, mostly smaller, but it all depends on which one is pinching at the time. These include mouth sores, "mouth blindness" — taste alterations or loss of sense of taste, also known as *dysgeusia* which is probably where the word "disgusting" came from — depression, fatigue, early menopause the list is endless.

My chemo regimen included three drugs: methotrexate and 5-fluorouracil taken by mouth, and cyclophosphamide, the real heavy that was administered by intravenous. This is a standard mix, used in the treatment of breast cancer throughout North America, depending on the stage of the disease.

Cyclophosphamide, or cytoxan, as it is also known, is one of the first generation of cancer drugs, a disturbing thought since chemotherapy has been around for a long time. The possibility of the use of cyclophosphamide in the treatment of cancer was the serendipitous result of an explosion on a ship carrying nitrogen mustard gas at the end of World War II. Many of the sailors exposed to the gas subsequently died of bone-marrow poisoning, a fatally low level of white blood cells. Someone figured that if this chemical destroyed fast-growing white blood cells, it would attack fast-multiplying cancer cells in a similar fashion.

Eureka. This "inadvertent experiment with chemical warfare" (Sontag, p. 65) put cancer patients into the front lines, like those caged canaries used to detect noxious gases in mines. A dead canary was the signal to abandon the mine shaft. However, cancer patients can't get out of the mine that fast. This drug is certainly not the first to be nearly as damaging as the disease it is supposed to eradicate.

Most chemotherapy damages the body's immune system because at the same time as it is wiping out cancer cells, it is

That Other Place

also suppressing the bone marrow which manufactures the white blood cells. That is why doctors keep such close tabs on a patient's white blood cell count and will not administer treatment if the count is too low. Often, blood transfusions are given to bolster the white blood cells before treatment can continue. Everyone I know who has had, or is having, chemotherapy treatment has had treatments postponed for this reason.

The importance of dosages and close monitoring cannot be overemphasized. "The patient must have luck on her side, a brilliant oncologist who administers the drug in exactly the right dosages and at the right time. But the whole treatment might fail because it strips the body of exactly what it needs to combat the disease in the first place." (Chopra, p. 46)

The ambivalence of chemotherapy is that at the same time as it is combatting cancer, it weakens the patient, knocking out the immune system and throwing down the ramparts for other diseases, including other forms of cancer. "In some cases — as high as 30% in breast cancer — new cancer appears, and the patient dies." (Chopra, p. 47)

When I started treatment though, I was much more worried about the more publicized side-effects of chemotherapy. At the clinic I was given information sheets listing what I might expect with each of the three drugs prescribed. For each drug, bone marrow depression was right up there, but since I had no idea what it meant, my glazed eye jumped to the more familiar and more graphic items, such as vomiting, tarry stools and hair loss.

Methotrexate
Most common:
   -low blood counts or bone marrow depression
   -nausea and vomiting
   -mouth and lip sores
   -loss of appetite
   -black tarry stools, bloody urine

Less common:
- hair loss (could be more frequent depending on dosage of drug)
- skin rash
- cough, shortness of breath
- dizziness, drowsiness, confusion
- headache
- joint pain
- swelling of feet or lower legs
- yellowing of eyes or skin.

5-fluorouracil
Most common:
- heartburn
- diarrhoea
- low blood counts and bone marrow depression
- skin rashes
- fatigue
- loss of appetite

Less common:
- nausea and vomiting (stomach should settle in 24 - 48 hours)
- mouth or lip sores
- black tarry stools
- stomach cramps
- dizziness, weakness
- hair loss

Cyclophosphamide
Most common:
- low blood count or bone marrow depression
- loss of hair
- loss of appetite
- nausea and vomiting (should settle down after 12 hours)
- painful urination, bloody urine
- missed menstrual periods
- taste changes

That Other Place

Less common:
  -cough, shortness of breath
  -dizziness, mental confusion
  -skin rashes

The winter ahead did not look promising.

After reading these lists, I expected to be bald, throwing up in all directions, mentally and physically incompetent, covered with sores, coughing and aching within a week. But slowly through the fog of fear came a little thought — I don't have to have *all* the side-effects. No need for greed.

As it turned out, I didn't have them all. But for the few I missed, I came up with others that weren't even on the list. My eyes dried out. Since no one told me this was a possible though fairly rare side-effect, I did not realize it was the result of chemo. I merely thought that besides having cancer, I was going blind. My eyes were so dry, they scraped when I rolled them. They were red, sore, puffy and UGLY.

"Oh, my dear, you'll need something for those eyes," said the oncologist at my weekly check-up. "You have a bad case of chemo-eyes."

What a relief. Chemo-eyes. She gave me three different prescriptions over the next few months and none of them worked. However, the condition cleared up by itself a few weeks after the last treatment. Only to come right back with radiation treatments. It wasn't an acknowledged side-effect of that treatment either. There were a lot of unacknowledged side-effects of both treatments, I discovered. Cynicism. Anger. Fear. Resignation. And a creeping, barely acknowledged hope that they work.

-XI-
Chemotherapy Fallout #1: Hair

Chemotherapy — Treatment using drugs to kill or damage cancer cells. Chemotherapy drugs usually act by inhibiting cell division ... Besides damaging cancer cells, chemotherapy drugs also damage healthy cells. But healthy cells recover more quickly than cancer cells...

Canadian Breast Cancer Series, Book Five

Bald: a host of associations is conjured by the bald or stubbled head of a woman. Despite Sigourney Weaver and Sinéad O'Connor, bald is not a popular fashion statement. The images are too strong, the associations atavistic and tremoring through our subconscious — a shaven head is disgrace, punishment, an emblem of being cast out, a sign of moral wrongdoing. The shaven heads of the women who fraternized with the enemy during World War II, the images of children in grey canvas shifts, their heads shorn against disease or nits, their eyes shining with a disgrace they do not understand. The sad powerful image in Seamus Heaney's poem, "Punishment":

> her shaven head
> like a stubble of black corn
> her blindfold a soiled bandage,
> her noose a ring
> to store
> the memories of love.
> Little adulteress,

> before they punished you
> you were flaxen-haired,
> undernourished, and your
> tar-black face was beautiful.
> My poor scapegoat,
>   ... (*North,*)

Bald. How do you cope with sudden and total baldness, especially rough for a woman but tough also for a man? You wear scarves, a wig, a toque, a dashing hat. But you still have to see yourself bald even if no one else does. Starting each day facing a bald person in the mirror is not getting the day off to a good start.

After my first treatment I waited with a kind of horrified fascination for my hair to fall out. I even tugged at it to see if it was loose. When it started to give way I was no longer fascinated. My stomach took a sickening lurch the first time a fistful of hair came out in the shower.

You are advised to be gentle. After that first handful I decided to be just the opposite. In a kind of frenzy to get it over with I tugged and brushed and pulled what seemed like pounds of hair from my head. And then it stopped coming out. This happened after each treatment. I began to believe that by treating it roughly, I was strengthening my hair and that was the very reason it was not all coming out.

Later I found that I was not alone in this approach. A friend from the cancer clinic had done much the same thing and had not lost all her hair either, although a year later she still feared waking up one morning to find it all on the pillow beside her shining scalp.

That's two cases. If I were a statistician I could build a statistic on that.

I had another technique, entirely secret, but I offer it now because it helped. I clenched my head. Nuts, right? Maybe, but in some sleepless midnight hours I swear I could make my skull tighten around the hair roots. It seems that such activities as head clenching are visualization techniques, a whole new world

Chemotherapy Fallout #1: Hair

I knew nothing about yet. At the time, thinking my hair on gave me a toehold on controlling at least one aspect of my life.

I did not lose all my hair. After each intravenous treatment, great hanks came out in the shower, festooning my body like spanish moss on an old tree. But I started out with such a thatch that I still had a thin covering at the end of chemotherapy. Although my hair changed in texture from strong, dark rather coarse curly hair to fine, wispy, grey, mouldy hay, I still had enough to gel into shape. That was a victory over the odds.

Before chemotherapy started, I was advised by the oncologist to buy a wig just in case. She said that it would give me a kind of security in being prepared should I wake up one day bald. People tend to go two quite different ways when the threat of baldness is thrust upon them. There are those brave creatures who say, "Right, now I can choose the hair I've always wanted," and pick a long curly blonde mane to wear over their fast-disappearing lanky mousy-brown wisps. And then there are the others, less adventuresome, who need the security of the familiar. They choose a wig that looks as much like their own hair and style as possible, no matter how much they thought they hated it. They may have spent years ironing their determined curls or curling their dead straight locks, but when it comes to the crunch they cling to the familiar. I was one of these.

On a Saturday morning, a couple of weeks after coming out of hospital and before chemo started, I went to the wig shop. I told no one where I was going. Partly it was the fear of taking this tangible step toward baldness: in going to the wiggery I was accepting the reality of what was about to happen to me. It was a frightening and — for some reason — shameful step. Why the shame? I don't know, but I obviously wasn't alone in this feeling. The wig shop was called Natural. Natural what? That was the point. It could be natural foods, natural brick or an environmentally conscious group bent on saving the ozone layer. The proprietor, a lovely young woman with a head of hair you could kill for, told me that she had left the word "wig" out of her business name because her clients did not like to be seen coming into a wig shop.

That Other Place

I did not exactly slink in, but I did check the street to see if anyone was watching. This nonsense reminded me anew of how surreal was my new world. The young owner was very reassuring, very sympathetic and very beautiful, tough to take when you have just had bits of your body removed, are preparing to lose more, and are feeling close to a hundred, thin and ugly. I eyed her tousled mane of hair to see if it were a wig. It was not.

We looked at books of pictures of different hair styles. It was like checking through magazines at the hairdresser's to choose a hair cut, but not as much fun. Unfortunately they all looked like wigs to me. In desperation I chose a rather classy brunette style that might have suited me ten years ago. Or maybe even two months ago.

A few days later the shop phoned my office and left a message. "Tell Ms. Williams that her Item has arrived."

A telephone call wrapped in plain brown paper guaranteed to throw the message-taker into a paroxysm of suspicion. Not at my office though, at that time a two-person operation, myself, reduced to an almost non-person, and my friend and colleague Pat Hood, who kept us going that whole rudderless year, I think through sheer willpower.

I went in to try on the Item and burst into tears. It was a lovely wig, no question. The problem was not the wig but the face beneath it. I felt like an old hag trying to fool the world and myself that I was still alive and kicking.

The Item was purchased and tucked away in a bureau drawer where I am delighted to report it has stayed ever since. Even though my own hair grew sparser and sparser, with first a glint, then a positive glow of skull showing through, and even though it turned greyer by the minute, even though it cracked rather than curled, even though what was left of it straightened into a kind of picture-mould around the ceiling of my head — it was mine own.

A word of advice: if you have to buy a wig for health reasons, ask your doctor to write a prescription for it. This usually ensures that the purchase price of it is covered by medical plans that include the cost of prescription drugs. It should be described as a prosthesis, which in a very real way it is.

For most people, loss of hair is devastating, not to be downplayed. The hearty "at-least-you-are-alive" admonitions of well-meaning friends are cold comfort for those people already dealing with misery-overload. Although in most cases there is no physical pain associated with hair loss (on occasion the scalp can become infected), its psychological effect is cruel. Your self-identity is already under attack without the disfiguring indignity of losing your hair. And not just on your head; pubic hair, eyelashes, eyebrows, body hair can all disappear. It usually all grows back. That is little consolation at the time.

A good wig allows you to pretend to be yourself. It is the camouflage that lets you move through the jungle of the normal world without pitying eyes piercing your disguise.

Even though men can be bald with impunity, unwanted baldness can be equally shattering for them as for women. One man I knew of shaved his head before starting treatment — so there would be no surprises, no hope crushed. When Bernie Siegel shaved his head, suddenly his patients started to open up to him, to tell him things they would never have discussed with him before because now they perceived him as a fellow traveller; he had a visible affliction. He has kept his head shaved ever since, as a symbol of empathy, keeping open the lines of communication.

Another man, who had just started chemotherapy, simply threw up and took to his bed for days after all his hair fell off in the shower. It just all let go at the same time. His wife got to clean the tub.

It is a strange and bizarre sensation to feel your hair letting go. Once, I thought a fly had settled on my head; I swiped at it, and a chunk of hair fell to the floor. There was no fly.

Pamela, my friend who tried to go through the five stages of dying in the right order even if it killed her, lost every hair on her head within two and a half weeks of starting treatment. When I met her, she was wearing a very pretty, curly silver-tipped wig that suited her beautifully. Since I had not known her

That Other Place

before, it looked absolutely right to me. Not to her though. When I commented on how good she looked, she was disbelieving. Her bright brave smile faded into a look of ineffable sorrow. She was looking from the inside out where the view wasn't as good.

However, Pamela was also the woman who announced one evening, "When I am through with chemo, I am going to be better. Then I am going to get a new wig and a new boyfriend. In that order." Her voice rang with defiance and with knee-jerk response I touched wood for her. There she was, utterly beaten about the ears with a Christmas diagnosis of lymphoma, surgery before New Year's, weekend hospital intravenous treatments, "lost weekends" once a month from which she would haul herself back to work by the following Tuesday. She was also on a steroid which had puffed her body up well beyond the compass of her wardrobe. Although she mostly wore a smile on her newly plump face, her eyes reflected the pain and bewilderment of her predicament.

She had recently lost a close member of her family to cancer, she still had radiation treatments to face, they had detected another tumour, but she was going to get a new wig and a new boyfriend. I wanted to hug her. A fellow traveller who, every time she was knocked off the road, scrambled back out of the ditch and continued on her journey.

When she died, less than three months later, many were convinced that it was the chemo, not the cancer, that had killed her.

-XII-
Chemotherapy Fallout #2: Nausea, Up, Down and Sideways

Chemotherapy is, to me, an indication of the sorry state of cancer treatment.

Eleanor Bergholz, "Under the Shadow of Cancer"

What a bland word, "nausea," from the Greek word *naus* meaning ship, originally meaning seasickness. Its definition has come to be much more specific: "sickness of the stomach, esp. when accompanied by a loathing for food and an involuntary impulse to vomit."

Well yes, but that is only the beginning. First of all, it is not necessarily just the stomach, it can be your whole entire being. At about my fourth treatment, in a vain attempt to get the feeling under control, I tried to go through it and by so doing, reach some kind of acceptance of it. I wrote down a description of exactly how I felt: "The nausea is a visible, tangible entity now, a malevolent creature that has taken up residence in my throat. It is a dead/live thing, a lump of sweet, putrefying, wet decay, a small animal with matted stinking fur, an evil malignant presence. Although it's dead, I taste its foul breath when I breathe."

During the first month of treatment, I felt mildly sick, very tired on the days of, and the first day after, each of the treatments at the clinic. But nothing much to speak of. Elation. I was going to be one of those people whose response was strong and controlled. No nausea for me. So when Dad, who had been ill for several weeks with a mysterious and painful ailment, said let's go to Florida for a few days, I said sure. What a mistake that was.

We should not have been allowed out on our own, Dad and I. To exercise my nearly strengthless right arm I tried swimming lengths in the ocean; the lengths became ever-decreasing circles; I was like a ship with its rudder locked. When I wasn't spluttering around on these dizzying laps, I was driving white-knuckled down the state freeways taking Dad anywhere but where we were. He wanted to go to the Everglades when we were at the seaside, and to the sea when we got to the Everglades. He wanted to be where his body wasn't. The Florida freeways were no escape route from his pain.

Dad spent nearly a month in hospital as soon as we got back home, finally having convinced the hospital staff (with the help of my doctor niece) that his pain was real. He had a severe but treatable arthritic condition that strikes without warning and, if undetected, can cause blindness and then death. Our mini-holiday had not worked for either of us. It was simply a reminder that there were to be no "Floridas" in our countries for a while.

At the beginning of chemotherapy, the clinic had asked if I would be part of a survey of the various psychological effects of the treatment. After my experience with Blitski/Blotski, the Talking Brain, I was wary of studies but agreed at least to talk to the student in charge. He was a compassionate young man, on the absolute opposite end of the spectrum from The Brain. He spoke of his mother who had had cancer since he was four years old. Because cancer was a context he had grown up in, he felt that he could sympathize but not really empathize with people whose diagnoses blast into families like lightning. I was just pathetically grateful to hear about anyone in the real world who had lived as long as his mother had, with breast cancer.

One of the questions on his survey, which he would ask me before each treatment, was, "Do you suffer from anticipatory nausea?" I didn't know what it was at first. I grew to know it intimately. Before the last two treatments, I was sicker the night before than I was the night after the intravenous. Wave after wave of sickness would sweep over me as treatment day came closer. I couldn't mention the clinic or treatment to anyone without choking back bile. Tears sprang from nowhere. Two days before treatment, Allen asked me what time my appointment was so that he could arrange to take me. Without warning I nearly drowned him in a great gust of weeping, as much of a surprise to me as to him. It was my body exercising its prerogative to be nothing but a physical storehouse for memory.

It was a revelation to me that chemo sickness could be cumulative. No one warned me although I asked the oncologists often about the possibility. They always were evasive, not through dishonesty but because they truly cannot predict with accuracy how chemo affects each individual patient. If they had cautioned me, what good would it have done? None, I guess. But as I got sicker with each treatment, I also got more resentful. Had I been warned I might have handled it better.

The second chemotherapy treatment was in November, a week after the disastrous Florida trip. I was a little more tired, a little sicker. A sense of fragility and depression clouded the days. But it was important to keep working, to keep living a normal existence, to fool everyone including myself that this major journey my life had become was merely a detour. Just another item to deal with. No dramatics. No self-important whining and whinging. What a crock. It was Allen who had to deal with the quivering mess that was me when the mask slipped.

My third treatment was to have begun on December 23, a date chosen by a sadistic nurse or fate. During those months, they often appeared to be the same to me, exercising the same inexorable unchallengeable force. But I inadvertently discovered that you did not have to lie down in front of the steamroller of fate.

As the treatment day grew near, I became less convinced that chemotherapy was the answer. I came up with all sorts of excuses why it was NOT a good idea to start again two days before Christmas, in the middle of my sister-in-law's visit from England, the day my kids were flying to Ireland to spend Christmas with their Dad, always a day fraught with anxiety. I have to fly them the whole way, each visit, get them past snarly attendants, uncaring ground staff, bombs, terrorists, Atlantic storms, drunken pilots, iced wings, sudden downdrafts ... It is a tough job, doing all this from the living room perched by the phone waiting to hear that they have arrived safely. Past trips have had me lurking over the instrument for days, wringing my hands and ringing Dublin every half hour.

I phoned the cancer clinic: please would it be all right to delay treatment for one week? Much humming and hawing. OK, the doctor says, one week. An hour later the clinic called back with a new appointment schedule that gave me a two-week delay. Two weeks? Why? No one knew. Back to the doctor.

Another phone call from the clinic staff: "Mrs. Williams, would you rather start treatment a week earlier?" No, I WOULD RATHER NEVER START TREATMENT AGAIN. What did they mean, would I like to start treatment? Did they mean *I* had a choice in this? Was it not carved in a medical stone tablet somewhere?

Of course I did not say any of this. My first Rule of Cancer: be nice to the clinic staff. Bake them cookies, buy their Christmas raffle tickets, drink their Tang in styrofoam cups and smile. Better to antagonize the Styx River boatman than these folks.

In the old country, from where I'd come, which I had never asked to leave, whose borders there was absolutely no problem crossing, I had been in control, sort of. I got up in the morning, had a cup of coffee, decided what to wear, where to go, how to deal with the day that was in it.

In this new country, my morning decisions suffered a sea change. The regimen of treatment put paid to any residual free will. Instead of deciding to fly to Denver (I've never been to Denver, but I always think of it as a place where decisive people live, or at least visit), I got to decide which hand to sneak out from under the bedclothes to grab a soda cracker, stealthily so that my brain would not recognize what my body was doing. Otherwise I would throw up before I could down a Stemital® or six, the anti-nausea drug I would have killed for.

It was the looming dearth of these pills that caused my first real altercation with the clinic staff. The receptionist was tired and cranky when I phoned about renewing the prescription.

Chemotherapy Fallout #2: Nausea, Up, Down and Sideways

"You get that from your family doctor," she intoned, just like the telephone operator in *Sorry Wrong Number*, the one who, with a bad case of terminal nasal drip, says, "You may diayayayal thahyt number direct, Murray Hill niyiyine, niyiyine, niyiyine niyiyine" while the murderer is sneaking up the stairs to dispense with the poor woman in the wheelchair. When you are on chemotherapy, without Stemital® or its equivalent, you feel a lot like that woman, with the muffled footsteps of the mad stabber at your back.

I got the drug after a steely-voiced conversation that included only a few of the things I would do to this poor kid on reception if she didn't manage to find a doctor to send me the prescription immediately.

Chemo was beginning to flatten my immune system, just as I had been warned at the start but had not understood; it was now attacking all the fast-growing cells besides cancer — hair follicles, the cells that line the digestive system, mouth and eyes — and the white blood cells responsible for fighting off infection. The discussion over just when I might start my third treatment was made academic by first a severe cold, then flu bordering on pneumonia. Chemo was out of the question until all these minor slings and arrows were cleared up, except I guess they weren't so minor, since apparently treatment is rarely postponed for anything less than "significant toxicity."

The doctors don't like postponing treatment, not because of any bureaucratic love of scheduling but because for metastatic breast cancer (indeed, for any metastatic cancer) it is essential to hit it as hard as possible and with no letup. "Attempting to be 'kind' to a patient by making toxicity as tolerable and minimal as possible can decrease the chances of a good result from the treatment. The kindest thing a physician can do is make sure the dose is as close to the theoretical maximum safe dose as possible and is also given on time." (Dollinger *et al.*, p. 253) My physicians were usually kindness personified.

The third treatment finally started in mid-January. I had done everything, short of dying, to avoid it. By the time I sat in the treatment chair, I was caught fast in the grip of anticipatory nausea. My mouth ran with saliva, I sweated, my eyes even sweated, at the thought of the first belt of chemicals in the vein. Yet, and this is puzzling, the first two sets of treatment didn't actually hurt; I didn't mind the needle in those earlier days; I don't mind new nurses; I had not been violently sick. What was it then, that was triggering this response? No idea. I just know that it was real and rough.

With anticipatory nausea came association nausea. About halfway through chemotherapy I met one of the chemo nurses in the meat section of a local supermarket. I smiled, said hello and clamped a hand over my mouth to keep from throwing up all over the chicken parts. It was the association of this really very nice woman with the therapy room. Abandoning my cart full of groceries, I beat a hasty retreat to the car. I hope that she, and all the chemo nurses in the world, have unshakeable self-confidence and realize that such violent reaction from their patients is not personal. It is simply Pavlov in the suburbs.

Except for the first treatment, a close friend or Allen came with me each time. This was of paramount importance. I made all the right noises, "No I don't need anyone to come, really I am fine," but I came to rely on them utterly — for company, for physical support, for laughter, real belly-aching laughter in the waiting room amidst the pain and fear and hope that permeated the very walls of that room.

One January day when I went on my own for blood tests only, and had forgotten my book, I studied my fellow travellers. There were 14 people in the waiting room, mostly in pairs. The trick was to figure out which one was the patient. With some it was no challenge: no hair, black eyes and canes were all clues that day. Sometimes though, the friends or spouses appeared to be in worse shape than their companions.

Each person has their own way of waiting. That day, one woman, not old, sat in a large chair, not so much sat as paused in the chair, her face a study of resignation, her movements slow, her eyes roving unseeing over the room. One hand rested open on her knee, the other curled loosely around the strap of her handbag. She was not hanging onto life any more. She was only

Chemotherapy Fallout #2: Nausea, Up, Down and Sideways

going through the motions.

There were the readers; they sat side by side, reading hard. Perhaps they were husband and wife but I was not clear which was the patient, which the "support person." Their eyes flicked up and darted back to the page each time the nurse called someone into the treatment rooms. They blocked reality with the printed page, taking Garrison Keillor's advice to seek out reality ... and deny it.

Then there were the talkers; they sat, head bent to head, murmuring, deep in conversation, apparently oblivious to the surroundings. They could have been at a chic little restaurant in the Market, gossiping over a salad and a glass of white wine. Their conversation sometimes was punctuated with laughter, sometimes with tears. The others in the room averted their faces from both. Either emotion seemed to be an intrusion.

On treatment days I was one of these people — fearful, hurting, all of that. But I was also insulated from my own thoughts and protected from the defeated ambience of the whole place by the chatter, the companionable silence, the very physical presence of Allen, Andy or Lucy.

The trauma of one treatment was completely erased by the worry that Andy, not I, was going to faint when the chemo nurse hooked me up to the intravenous. Andy turned resolutely to the wall, swaying dangerously when she caught sight of the needle. "I'm right here if you need me," she said to the refrigerator she had her face buried in. It was exactly the sort of help I needed. Doubled up with laughter sure beat being doubled up with pain. With Lucy, one day in the waiting room, a yellow-coated cancer society volunteer interrupted our conversation to offer Lucy a cup of tea and a cookie. She pointedly ignored me. I loved it, thinking that she had mistaken me for a too boisterous "support person." On reflection, I realized that she was pointedly ignoring me so that she wouldn't have to deal with what I might have done with her tea and cookie. They wouldn't have matched the rug ...

A later treatment, the toughest of all, was made bearable because Allen was there to hang on to; when the drugs hit me, I tried to flee the onslaught, the wave of a weird excruciating invasion that had found the very core this time; the only thing that kept me anchored in the chair and still attached to the goddam tubes was the warmth and comfort of Allen's presence. In the grinding grey seas of chemo, I clutched his hand in a bruising grip to keep from drowning.

Somewhere around the fourth treatment I got sick again, with flu and a cold, all the usual stuff that Canadian winters are made of. I paid no heed. However, I hadn't fully grasped the danger of exposure to even minor errant germs, armed against them with an immune system that was going down for the third time. And it wasn't waving but drowning. Like a prize fighter at the end of each round, flattened on the canvas, you get your blood counts from the referee.

I felt a tremendous ambivalence toward these counts. On the one hand, I was pleased when the white blood cells were showing signs of withstanding the chemo; it meant that they were there fighting cancer too. On the other hand, if the counts were low, it meant that chemo treatments had to be deferred. It was the short term versus the long term. And somewhere in those winter months the short term wrestled the long term to the ground and stood triumphant. I cheered aloud, right there outside the chemo room, when a nurse came to tell me there would be no treatment that day since my blood counts were way too low.

I was out of there like a missile, and home to enjoy dinner, made by Sue. She brought dinner over every treatment day throughout all those months, another rope of the net that kept me from hitting bottom through the dark days.

But low blood counts and cancelled treatments just prolonged the process. I didn't actually get to skip any; they were just added on at the end. That day though I remember the euphoria at avoiding the chemo room and the delight of the nurse delivering the message; my shortsightedness was contagious, and I was grateful for her supportive glee at my reprieve.

As the six months of treatment extended to seven and then stumbled into the eighth month, the long-term perspective struggled up from the canvas. The day of my expected last

Chemotherapy Fallout #2: Nausea, Up, Down and Sideways

treatment I had been turned away again. I had told anyone who would listen that it was to be my LAST treatment. Saying LAST like that, right out loud, attracted the attention of those damn gods again, those capricious, malicious creatures waiting to confound anyone who has designs on the future. Like me. I was starting to make plans to live it again.

I was sent away without treatment and this time I was not gleeful. Please, God, I just wanted it over.

The oncologist had warned me that when it was finished, I should be prepared for a downtime; that I wouldn't necessarily feel elated and happy that it was over. It was a gentle sort of by-the-way caution. I heeded it only to the extent that I was sure that it wouldn't apply to me. At that moment I was living only for the end of chemotherapy. If an extra treatment had been added, I could not have stood it, so carefully had I parcelled out my meagre supply of endurance. It was inconceivable that I would not be over the moon the very day of my last visit to the chemo room at the clinic.

Finally the day came. The nurses were full of good cheer: "Your last treatment — congratulations!" I wished them goodbye, cheerfully announcing that I never never wanted to see any of them again and wobbled off on the arm of Lucy who took me home and badgered me into bed. Those hours after treatment not only passed in a blur now, they were completely lost time. I had no memory of reading the mail, talking on the phone, whatever got in the way of me and bed. That last day, pole-axed as usual, I collapsed waiting for the good feelings to roll on.

May 1989
Sylvia and I sat on our front door step, soaking up the early spring sun that held the faintest whisper of summer warmth to come. Sylvia looked wonderful, her face glowed.

"I've never felt better," she said. "Here I am, after 25 years of stomach problems, back problems, husband problems, and I feel wonderful. Do you know, I think I've had this for all that long."

"This" was ovarian cancer. It was a year after her surgery and diagnosis, a year in which she had carved her own way through the rock-hard conventions of treatment of her disease.

We had both just returned from the cancer clinic, from check-ups, blood tests, each on our own route, but sharing the journey.

Her doctor had told her that day that she could no longer stay on the mild chemotherapy regimen she'd been following for the year — pills she claimed had no more side-effects than aspirin. However, they apparently had a cumulative effect which could result in leukemia. What a fellow with ovarian cancer did not need was leukemia.

"So what can they give you?" I asked, still in the thraldom of doctors as God and the magic bullet syndrome.

"Nothing," Sylvia answered with serenity. "They suggested radiation. Maybe, maybe not. We'll see. Right now, I am just enjoying life."

The dragon sat between us on the steps, his scaly arms draped around our shoulders.

We ignored him, the warming earth and budding trees our guarantee of a future which did not include him.

-XIII-
Only a Pause on the Journey

Breast cancer likes to come back in the liver, lungs and bones.
Oncologist, Ottawa Civic Hospital

They didn't. Seaton and Sue arrived with champagne and flowers later that week to celebrate. Chemo was finished. So was I, nearly, but it was over. I stayed at the Banff Springs Hotel for a few sybaritic days while Allen attended some meetings. The weather was crisp and glorious, the mountains snapped and sparkled in the spring air. I walked along the Bow River into the village — and had to take a taxi back. I said how fine I felt, but I lied. What excuse did I have for not feeling wonderful? I felt guilty that elation had not arrived on schedule, only a miasma of ill-ease, of weariness, of vague depression. Now what?

In some perverse way the visits to the clinic and the chemo treatments had become a tortured security blanket. Now without them I felt cast adrift back in the old world without any protection against the enforced new perspective. I had lost the fit to my old life. Surely it was simply a matter of time before I was reeled back across the border again, because wasn't I just visiting? After so many months of major wrenches and adjustment, "that other place" had more reality than all the years of living gone before. Here was a conundrum.

At the end of chemotherapy two things deepened the depression. One was the persistent feeling that I was letting everyone down because I wasn't feeling great and — more important — NORMAL. You've had surgery, you've finished your treatment, you are still alive, you have no overt signs of recurrence, so now get back to your life. Put it all behind you. Be normal. It was just a detour. Stop snivelling about what's passed and get on with it. Not one person actually said that to me but I still felt guilty as hell because I couldn't.

And the other distress was that it seemed everything I read now offered authoritative proof that not only did chemo not work, it actually caused cancer. The knife edge of such research sliced any tender shoots of optimism that I might really be able to turn in my passport to the world of the sick and frolic back into the sunlight of good health. "It is one of the tragic ironies of modern cancer treatment that while attacking the cancer, the treatments usually attack the body's own immune defences. Malignant tumours are continually changing and throwing off seeds (metastases) which are difficult to detect and harder to treat. The patient needs every ounce of immunity during treatment, to mop up these seeds and to act against leftovers of the original tumour. Therefore by reducing the strength of immunity, chemotherapy and radiotherapy can actually promote the spread of the cancer." (Fuldor, p. 115)

Well, sheeeeit. What do I do now? I couldn't back up, start over and take another route.

At Banff, when I was struggling with the realization that nirvana was not happening the way it was supposed to, I read that "The tremendous disadvantage [of chemotherapy] is that the whole body is damaged in the assault on one of its parts. In the case of chemotherapy, there is the very real danger that the immune system will become so weakened that the door is opened for other cancers to develop in the future. However, untreated breast cancer is considered deadly, and today's medicine is good at wiping it out *over the short run* [my emphasis]." (Chopra, p. 14)

At my own connivance had I aided the disease by agreeing to take these toxic drugs? Was chemo a form of suicide? Would it just finish off what cancer had started?

It was a while before I realized, and finally, finally, it was a comforting, strengthening realization, that if I could go back and choose again I would choose the same course. It was the right one for me. Whatever happens. Since then I've met many people with cancer for whom chemo was not the right choice — because they did not choose to take it. Françoise, a vibrant young woman with deep brown eyes that shone with commitment to her own way, refused chemotherapy after a lumpectomy which ousted the malignant tumour and three infected lymph nodes ... but not the cancer. Just under five years after her surgery, cancer was confirmed in her other breast and possibly in her spine.

"Non, merci," she said to the first oncologist who advised a full mastectomy this time, and heavy-duty chemo. Her face lit up when she recounted her defiance. Underneath the apparent china-like fragility of her body was a will of iron and a certainty that this was not the route for her. Despite other oncologists telling her the same thing, she did not heed them.

"I put a big X across chemo," she told me as we waited in the sunlight outside the church waiting for the funeral to begin. It was the third funeral in ten days for friends who had succumbed to cancer. "When the doctors told me, you have not two years to live, I put a big X across the doctors. It is not for them to tell me how long I can live."

I stood in awe of her courage. After the funeral she was going to a cabinet maker to have a special bed made, with a canopy and four posters. She was no longer able to work, she had little money left but she laughed with delight as she described the bed she would have. I don't know whether the new bed, meditation and visualization, vitamins and herbs will keep the cancer at bay longer than a few belts of chemo. Probably for her they will. But the question is academic, pernicious even. She has chosen her own treatment, and she is working *with* it, not against it in fear and loathing.

This same blessed two weeks, among the funerals, the grieving and the fear, a friend phoned me from out of town. Her breast cancer had come back and was apparently out of control. At the

That Other Place

first mastectomy site a huge open wound had developed — a nurse came every day to her home to change the dressing. "I don't understand it," she said, "here I am, so happy, happier than I've been perhaps ever. I can't believe what is happening to my body."

Her voice revealed her shaken faith in the mind/body connection upon which she had founded her battle against the disease.

"They want me to take chemo. I've never had it," she spoke softly. "I suppose I'll give it a shot, if only for the sake of my kids and J."

It is not for the sake of anyone but you, I wanted to shout. Just you. Don't just make the gesture. It won't work. But I didn't say any of this, coward that I am. Who was I to be giving advice? I am just another bewildered mouse in this maze.

I should have had more faith in my friend. She is far too clever to have sabotaged her own treatment with such negative feelings. She has been working with the chemotherapy treatments, which have been excruciatingly tough, but they are working. She has taken a giant step back from the edge and lives now with renewed hope and energy.

I don't think chemo will really work for a person who is dead set against it, who doesn't believe that it might help. There is too strong a connection between feelings and physical reactions to expect a physical treatment to work without the emotions cheering it on. If chemo is anathema to you, your mind/body is primed against the possibility of success. The war within becomes a war between you and the treatment rather than between you and the disease. "Oh, terrific," you say? "Another benighted guilt trip. If chemo doesn't work, it's all my fault. I am sabotaging success by not loving chemotherapy." Wrong. Better to fight the disease with weapons that you don't turn against yourself.

If you can stand chemo — if you can *with*stand chemo — then go for it if it is the treatment recommended by your doctors. There are so many degrees of treatment, so many individual responses, there is really no predicting the side-effects for each person. Statistically it is obviously a boon, successfully treating various cancers, and at various stages of the disease it accomplishes different things. For instance, it keeps the pain at bay when breast cancer has metastasized into the bones or organs. Do not reject it out of hand. Explore, ask questions, ferret out new treatments. Or get someone to do the research for you. Do not slam doors on any exits from "that other place."

-XIV-
Chemotherapy Fallout #3: Instant Menopause

Rumor has it that the menopausal woman is deranged, even criminal ...

Dickson and Henriques, *Women on Menopause*

It was becoming clear to me that the end of chemotherapy treatments did not mean the end of chemotherapy. There were the physical inroads the treatment itself had taken, not to be shaken off in a hurry. I remembered the pre-chemo days when I could walk further than the end of the lane without reeling with exhaustion, when I could brush my hair without apprehension, when I could eat something and actually enjoy it. And then there was this other legacy, another claw of the crab that was pinching with increasing ferocity: premature menopause.

The choice of drugs (there are more than 50 different chemo drugs) partially depends on what kind of tumour you have. In many cases, including mine, artificial menopause is one of the objectives of the treatment, not an inadvertent side effect. Tumours can be hormone-negative or hormone-positive; that is, the amount of estrogen or progesterone receptors in a tumour indicates its dependence on hormones for growth. Apparently it is a Better Thing, if you have a tumour at all, to have one that is hormone-positive because it is more likely to respond to hormonal treatment such as the drug, tamoxifen, which blocks

Chemotherapy Fallout #3: Instant Menopause

estrogen from stimulating the growth of cancer cells. Without the receptors, this drug is ineffective, thus eliminating a form of treatment that is proving to be effective for some breast cancers. "Tumours with positive receptors are associated with a better patient prognosis and longer survival." (Dollinger *et al.*, p. 253).

Mine was hormone-negative. That was one of the Bad News bulletins. The Good News was that I did not know that it was Bad News for four years after diagnosis and treatment, not because I wasn't told, but because I wasn't hearing properly. The negative-receptor aspect of my tumour was one of the reasons for initial aggressive treatment, because if there is a second time around, hormone therapy will not work. However, I had all this so thoroughly twisted, I thought it was better to be negative than positive (like the results of biopsies), and that my oncologist was trying to cheer me up when she told me this. The downside was, of course, that it was crucial for menopause to be induced, to reduce hormonal activity in my body.

My reaction to this was, so what? On a scale of one to ten, it was about two on my worry list. Too many other looming things to fret about. And besides, I thought, I'm closing in on it anyway, why fuss about an early start.

A year into menopause, I heard Vicki Gabereau on CBC radio interviewing Janine O'Leary Cobb, the author of a book on menopause and the editor of a newsletter on the subject. They were agreeing that menopause certainly had a bad press, practically a non-existent one until recently. Vicki said that it was tainted with death — that when women were no longer reproductive, they felt they were dying. Ms. Cobb said that for most women, menopause was a shameful subject, that they would happily own up to suffering from PMS but would not discuss being pre- or post-menopausal.

I joined the discussion ... in the privacy of my car, "Hey, listen, you guys," I said to my radio, "I know how you break the taboo. You get cancer, then you have chemotherapy, then if you are pre-menopausal, you aren't any more, you are instantly menopausal, a real treat but, hey, you don't worry about it anyway because in the overall scheme of things it ranks right down there with the hangnails." Tunnel vision, another side-effect of cancer and its treatments can have its moments, eliminating the minor slings in favour of the focus on Life's Large Events.

True though. In the midst of chemo, the hot flashes, freezing sweeps, the drenching sweaty tides queued up for attention. The Pollyanna in me chirped, "Pay no heed; at least they aren't life-threatening." And the depression; who knows from which of the many possible sources it came from.

At the time. Later, the menopausal stuff started to creep up the ladder of misery, although never as high as where the female population of California seems to have put it. "Women who are menopausal in California are around the bend — they view it like cancer." (Sheehy, p. 43) There we go again, the final bloody touchstone for the rest of the population.

Within days after my first treatment, the first wave of menopausal clues hit without warning: hot flashes, joint pain, fatigue, night sweating, freezing spells, crawly skin and maybe memory loss which has probably blocked out lots more horrors. And of course, no more periods. All these were the result of an immediate drop in hormone production.

Most women go through a peri-menopausal period, about ten years of creeping up on the real thing. During this time the ovaries secrete less estrogen but the body compensates by releasing more hormones from other sources. Those women who have had menopause brought on artificially, (through surgery, radiation, chemotherapy or disease) don't get to sneak up on it. There is no easing in, just wham, from one month to the next. Since there is no time for other sources of hormone production to kick in, it's a form of cold turkey. "The more abrupt the drop in estrogen, the more severe the symptoms." (Sheehy, p. 130)

The medical treatment for these various forms of "discomfort," the euphemism most often used to describe the effects of menopause, natural or induced, is hormone (or estrogen) replacement therapy. However, the jury is still out on HRT. The discussion seems to boil down to what you would prefer to die of. Combined with all the fear-mongering of estrogen therapy and cancer come other studies suggesting that estrogen for post-menopausal women could reduce risk of heart disease by as much as 50 percent. Here we are in Alice-in-Wonderland again: if cancer is your disease of choice, then take estrogen; if it's heart disease, then don't take it. Hobson, are you listening?

There are other deterrents to the worry-free gobbling of estrogen: one source lists the following as common side-effects of HRT: "nausea, weight gain, bloating, vaginal itching, breakthrough bleeding, and sore or tender breasts ... Some women ... develop high blood pressure." And here comes the kicker: "There is also an increased risk of developing cancer of the uterus, gallbladder disease, or blood clots." (Belisle, p. 3) But breast cancer? I wondered weakly.

After four years I still cannot find a book or doctor that can explain unequivocally the actual connection between breast cancer and hormone activity. There are discussions on hormone *treatment* after you have breast cancer but not on how hormones might cause cancer in the first place. In *The Silent Passage,* Gail Sheehy discusses the relationship between breast cancer and hormones and finds contradictions at every turn. "The risk of getting breast cancer rises steadily with age, after menopause, in *all* women, including those who are not secreting estrogen or taking it in replacement hormones — right up to the age of one hundred." (p. 118) "Studies that attempt to document any causative link between HRT [hormone replacement therapy] and breast cancer are doomed to be inconclusive ..." (p. 119) But, "The most complete review of studies on the estrogen-cancer link, recently reported by the Centres for Disease Control, found a direct linear relationship: For up to five years of using menopausal estrogen, no increased risk was found. But a woman who uses estrogen pills for fifteen years has a 30 percent greater risk of developing breast cancer." (*Ibid.*) A statement under the "risks" column about taking estrogen therapy sums up the dilemma for those of us who have/had breast cancer: "Unknown associations with breast cancer." (p. 129)

The data connecting hormone therapy to increased risk of uterine cancer seem to be more conclusive but the connection with breast cancer is fraught with other issues as well as conflicting research. Since some varieties of breast cancer tumours are classed as hormone-dependent, women with this kind of cancer should never take estrogen because it could stimulate the growth of cancer. But hormone-positive breast cancers are actually treated with hormone therapy, which gives them another kick at the can if cancer recurs.

Since hormone treatment was out for me, I asked my GP if there was anything else that might relieve the various nasty accoutrements of instant menopause. She was sympathetic but her basic message was "live with it." The unspoken corollary was "at least you are alive. It is a small price to pay." She gave me a pamphlet on menopause. (She was about 30 years old at the time.) In my work I have often edited and even written similar types of brochure. You try to put yourself in the reader's place to ensure that what you are saying is of some use. This brochure was quite well written, had interesting drawings, provided facts in several areas but offered only one miserable shred of advice for controlling the monstrous effects of artificially induced menopause without estrogen: "Modify your life style and diet." Thank you. This means giving up eating and drinking all your favourite things and boring yourself to death by running 10 miles a day, replacing hot flashes with ruined heels and arthritis of the knees and hips.

I gave up drinking coffee, which resulted in withdrawal headaches and absolutely no reduction in hot flashes, hot sweats, cold flashes, etc. I gave up drinking wine, with the same non-results except I didn't get headaches because I was drinking coffee again. I started to exercise more. At aerobics class the heat flashes had me sloshing around the gym, with my classmates maneuvering out of my sodden, slipping vicinity with increasingly frantic jumping jacks. The term "flashes" is totally inaccurate because it suggests speed; the heat builds with various forewarnings to an unbearable peak, lingers while you try to keep your brain from short-circuiting, then tails off in

Chemotherapy Fallout #3: Instant Menopause

a sweaty, prickly denouement. I have tried various remedies prescribed by my increasingly sympathetic GP (she's getting older now ...). None has helped.

So now I know why the books and brochures do not go into detailed advice for newly menopausal women with breast cancer, except don't become one. At this juncture in medical time, there is no antidote, nor is the search for one high on the list of medical priorities. One cryptic reference in Sheehy's book suggests that there might be something out there. A 37-year-old woman on chemotherapy was made instantly menopausal by the drug cytoxan which caused ovarian failure. "The untimely menopause caused her months of interrupted sleep and insomnia, along with mounting anxiety and feelings of depression ... Once the reason became clear [menopause] medication corrected the problem. (p. 79) HEY! What medication?? She doesn't say, but I continue to look in hope.

For the most part, however, reading such books as Sheehy's and Janine O'Leary Cobb's from the wrong side of cancer is totally demoralizing. You keep falling through the trap door of such phrases as, "Unless there are strong reasons for artificially menopausal women *not* to have it, estrogen replacement therapy is started almost immediately." (Belisle) Right, skip this section. The damn horse has already bolted from the barn and no amount of door slamming is going to put it back in. So you leap the chaff that tells you what to do to avoid getting cancer and search for the wheat that tells you how to live with it and the spectre of its recurrence. Drugs such as Provera® might help, but you must ensure that they are safe to take with whatever cancer you have/had. And there are some natural remedies that might ease some of the symptoms. Vitamin E, Vitamin B, acupuncture, sensible exercise, sensible diet ... so far I have not found a magic elixir that a) works and b) doesn't encourage cancerous growth. Let me be honest though. Perhaps if I stuck with a "no coffee, no alcohol, no sugar, no fats, no fun" routine and I exercised steadily and daily rather than in bursts of frenetic dedication interspersed with sloth, I might be more successful. At a dinner party I was complaining about how all these healthy antidotes were pretty much a crock. A friend said evenly, "You have to stop drinking coffee and wine for more than a day, you know." Rats, I knew there was a catch.

My friend, Sylvia, didn't even look for an alternative to HRT. She turned her back on the whole medical community when told that she must never take estrogen again. She had been on it for 20 years. For her, this no-hormone edict in itself was a death knell.

"What do you mean, no estrogen? You might as well say 'no more water",' she responded.

The wise doctor shook his ponderous head and waggled a godlike finger. "My dear, estrogen for you is out of the question. You are strong, you can do without it."

He probably then went home and knocked back a couple of martinis before dinner, martinis that of course he could do without but that he had been drinking for 30 years and would fight to the death if anyone said "No more martinis, doctor. You are strong. You can do without them."

This incident exactly mirrors an episode recounted by a woman doctor, Mathilde Krim, in Sheehy's book:

> [A] group of male physicians [were] discussing [a] woman's case; her cancer was of the lung. The patient was asked what other medication she took. "Estrogen," she volunteered.
> "That's the first thing to cut out," the men ordered.
> "Why, if it makes her feel better?" demanded Dr. Krim. "It was absurd. The poor woman had all the problems with her lung cancer, and now she had to suffer hot flashes on top of it." But the males physicians were gratuitously adamant. (p. 37)

It all depends on where you sit. For many doctors, the latest medical theories, whether or not backed up with scientific evidence, take precedence over the individual needs. So many medical edicts are based on passing theory, with no more scientific basis than my depression theory (see below).

Witness the about-faces that pepper medical history. Amputate, don't amputate. Take out tonsils at an early age, don't

Chemotherapy Fallout #3: Instant Menopause

take out tonsils unless they are so infected they separate the body from the head. Bleed the patient, throw out the leeches. Keep a new mother in bed for ten days drinking Guinness and eating peanuts, yank a new mother out of bed within hours of giving birth and send her home to deal with the reality of having a day-old baby, and probably a toddler or two, in her exhausted fragile care. Eat spinach, it builds up muscles and is *good* for you — generations of kids were bullied by Popeye into downing plates of green sludge. Now, don't eat spinach, too much iron will kill you. Have a mammogram every year from age 40; don't have a mammogram because a) they are misleading in pre-menopausal women and b) there is some evidence to suggest that too many mammograms *increase* the risk of breast cancer because of the amount of exposure to radiation. It all depends on the year, possibly the *politically* correct thinking of the moment.

So take estrogen and get cancer. Don't take it, and have a heart attack. Tails you lose; heads you lose.

For Sylvia, whose choice was made before many of these recent "findings" about estrogen were made public, estrogen was more important than living miserable years without it. Couldn't her doctor have listened more closely to her needs and tried to come up with a compromise or response that would have truly been ministering to her as a person — with stage 3 ovarian cancer — rather than trotting out the generic response so singularly unsuitable to her circumstances?

Of course doctors must be abreast of current medical thinking; they should also recognize when it is more important to abandon it than to follow it slavishly. And so should patients. Sometimes it is better to listen to your own instincts which are based on impeccable empirical research — your own body — than eclectic medical advice gleaned from an averaging based on statistics.

Women handle the onset of menopause, natural or artificially induced, in different ways. My sister-in-law and good friend whom I hadn't seen for a long time, told me in a long-distance, long overdue conversation about all the recent changes in her life. "Monumental," she said, "emotional, physical, intellectual ... a clean sweep. It's terrifying."

That Other Place

I sympathized, suggesting that some of these might be associated with menopause. But she didn't need sympathy. She was exhilarated by the change. "Perhaps it is menopause, but meno 'pause' is just that, isn't it? A pause not an end, a regrouping and gearing up for the next stage of life rather than the beginning of the slide into old age."

What a great attitude. I was full of admiration while struggling in the grip of a hot flash that had me sliding not into a new stage but out of my chair in a swoosh of sweat. "But what do you do about the hot and cold, the moods, the depression, the despair, the sore skin, all the nasty business of this pause?"

There was a silence, then her beautiful Welsh accent came lilting across the line — "Weeell, perhaps you must just ... adjust your clothing."

Boy, did that make me feel like a whiner. When the searing heat boils over you, accompanied with its tilt of despair, its slithery crawly sensation on the skin, its rolling wave of sweat preceded by a spell of freezing, just "adjust your clothing."

The temptation is to rip every stitch of clothing right off. I suppose that is a form of adjusting. This gentle instruction became my new motto; instead of plucking frantically at the neck of my sweater or shirt to let in a breath of cool air, I would whisper into the onslaught of heat, "Just adjust your clothing. Stop over-reacting." It didn't work.

During the winter nights of chemo, hot and cold flashes had me whirling like a rotisserie. To forestall a threatening wave of heat, I'd throw the bedclothes off fast, exposing my whole sweaty body to the Arctic winds whistling through the open window. And exposing the whole of Allen's shivering body as well. It is impossible to believe that people around you are not on the same roller coaster of temperature. When you are freezing, you bundle your partner's steaming body up with extra blankets; when you are baking, you pull the covers off anyone within arm's length.

All that winter and spring though, the fact that my thermostat had gone haywire didn't really bother me compared to chemotherapy. However, with the summer months, menopause symptoms soared to the top of the list, second only to radiation burn and fatigue.

No one had ever told me about cold flashes which, that summer in the middle of a 90-degree day, had me shivering and piling on sweaters, only to strip down to a panting minimum about five minutes later. I had to ask people what the weather was like while I was standing in it. My personal weather surrounded me like a shroud, distorting my view of the world.

There is a theory, explained to me by a doctor, about why menopause includes depression and anxiety. The hot flashes and flushes are similar to the body's response to embarrassment and fear under normal conditions. (For example, some people blush and heat up with embarrassment if they have to address a roomful of people.) When a menopausal hot flash starts to build up, your body reverses the association: the heat and sweat trigger the anxiety.

It isn't anxiety so much that gets to me, it is the despair, the few seconds of black desolation and hopelessness that heralds the onslaught of the heat. My own theory is that these little droplets of despair, over the months, wear a groove in the brain, like water dripping on rock, carving a route into the mind for deeper and more enduring depression later on.

The empirical research supporting this theory is drawn from a cohort of one — me. The corroborating secondary source research, which I read after developing my theory, consists of one sentence in Janine O'Leary Cobb's book: "The risk of depression is high for women [whose menopause has been artificially induced] with the incidence highest about two years after the operation [chemo or radiation]." (p. 10) These do not provide quite a broad enough sample to convince the medical community, but my theory is as sound as leeching and if I work at it, I could come up with a statistic ...

On menopause, either natural or induced, the underlying messages from the medical community are depressingly similar. Be glad you live in the late 20th century when your life expectancy is more than 50. Women in earlier centuries didn't have to worry a lot about menopause because so few of them made it to that stage in their lives.

Fine. I am thankful I live in the 20th century. In the 16th century the average life span was 35 years. In the 19th century it was about 45. And now it is 75 years. Why? Among other things, developments in medical knowledge. So, if medicine has helped women to reach menopause, how come it can't help us deal with it better?

One reason is that menopause, as doctors keep pointing out, is a relatively new phenomenon for the female population. Another is the lack of interest of a male-dominated medical community. Menopause is not up there in the front-runners for research funding. It is a stage in life, right? So you live it. And it's not our stage of life, so we'll get to it later.

Although this is beginning to change as the aging population makes its needs and interests felt, menopause is still a neglected condition, and often a vicious one. Not a disease, of course, but a part of a woman's life, however reached, which we have been programmed to grin and bear. Silently. Which is why we are still in the dark ages about how to alleviate the misery that often accompanies it.

-XV-
The Simons Hold a Tumour Board Meeting

When you come to the fork in the road, take it.

Yogi Berra

After the last of chemotherapy and the few shaky days at Banff, Allen and I went on a real holiday to mark my launch into the land of the well. We drifted down the Colorado River through the desert, a fine lazy time full of reading, swimming and sitting on the deck of a houseboat. In the evenings we watched the moon rise over the red rocky outcrops, and listened to the scuttling lizards and the squeaks of the tiny bats dipping through the sky.

Just before dawn as the moon slid below the horizon the stars blazed out in a final crescendo. It was all pretty perfect. And I could read omens and find symbolism everywhere. On a desert stroll one late afternoon, I nearly stepped on a rattlesnake that coiled and reared into attack mode in a flash. He became an indelible image of cancer lurking somewhere in my body ready to strike again. A less whimsical reminder was when I collapsed in the parking lot of a supermarket, almost fainting in a sweep of nausea and terror that chemo had merely postponed the inevitable.

An appointment with a radiologist was scheduled for when we returned home. It was a routine appointment, arranged by the oncologist to cover all the bases, to enlist the support of a second opinion that radiation was not on the cards for me. The second opinion was that I *should* have radiation therapy. Since in those days I was still clinging to the belief that doctors were gods, this was a shocker. Obviously the gods in this new place were like those loose cannons of Mount Olympus whose whimsical tyrannies created such havoc in the lives of mortals. I was truly havocked.

What happens when the Simons disagree right there in front of you, and all you want is for them all to tell you in confident tones the one Right Thing that you must do? If you follow their instructions, a happy ending comes with a guarantee, right? That is not how it works. I already knew that with part of my brain; this latest evidence put paid to any lingering trust in medical certainties.

The appointment with the radiologist began with a conversation with his resident. My previous experiences with residents were not such that I wanted to spend a lot of time with the breed. When Matt was born and I haemorrhaged and had to be rushed back to hospital, it was a resident who gave my blood transfusion to the wrong patient, probably already brim full of blood, while I lay all night on a rock-hard stretcher in the emergency department, "wan and paley loitering." It was a resident who frightened me almost right out of the hospital the night before surgery by insisting that I sign forms giving the surgeon permission to cut off anything he saw fit to remove while I was conveniently unconscious.

So I was on my guard when the radiation resident arrived. He was an exceedingly young man, apparently 9 or 10 at the most, and certainly it was beyond his bedtime. His hollow eyes and a tic in his cheek suggested severe sleep deprivation. He inched through the door on a huge yawn. His plaid, flared trousers were not reassuring: a doctor wearing flared trousers in 1989 probably was still practising 1960s medicine. Except that obviously he wouldn't have been born yet.

His total fatigue was evident in the boneless flapping of his wrists and in his eyes that fluttered shut between slurred phrases that never made it into a complete sentence. Meandering into a thicket of words, he would wave his hands helplessly in search of an exit. He'd drift to a stop, then suddenly

The Simons Hold a Tumour Board Meeting

yelp "yes" in schizophrenic agreement with whatever he was trying to say. He was the only one who understood enough to respond. I was flummoxed.

"You ... had ... um ... surgery ... um ... last year and I see you ... er ... have ... just finished .... chemotherapy ... um ... that was ... um .... Yes."

I waited. Yes what?

"And how ... um?"

"The chemo?" I prompted helpfully.

"Yes."

"Fine." I lied fast because he was obviously going to nod off before I finished speaking.

Silence.

Finally his eyes focused on me with a startled look. Where had I come from?

Nudging the conversation along, I asked, "Were my blood counts OK last visit? I forgot to ask."

"You keep ... um ... track ... er ... like ...?" His weariness was tinged with reproach.

"I do," I said, biting off the urge to justify. I didn't want to put his attention span to the test.

The pauses between his increasingly vague questions and my rapid-fire replies grew more pronounced, giving me time to wonder at the respective roles of patients and doctors. Whose responsibility was it to keep the social ball rolling, his or mine? Who was responsible for the direction of the conversation between the medical practitioner and patient? Guilt was starting to creep in. It was either up to me to liven things up and keep this guy interested, or let the poor sod sleep.

The conversation jerked along when suddenly his words blistered into my consciousness. I was so intent on keeping things moving, I had stopped trying to make sense of what he was saying.

"A tumour .... um ... yours .... that .... um ... er.... you know .... negative receptors ... um Yes. Less ... um ... likelihood ... er ... survival ... Yes. I mean ... statistics say ... um ... but for each individual ... Yes! It might not be ... of recurrence of ... um ...Yes."

He obviously agreed with himself, but if I had understood him correctly, not with my oncologist.

Less likelihood of survival? I thought I had been told more, but that in the event of returning cancer, hormone therapy could not be used — that was the bad news. Sleepy here had turned everything on its ear, pronouncing, between snoozes, that my kind of tumour had been of a fast-growing, virulent variety. *That* was the bad news. The shreds of comfort I had derived from earlier explanations from the oncologist apparently had been of my own concoction and withered before Sleepy's lazy blast of reality.

I had been comforting myself with apples and, like Snow White, discovered that apples were not something to mess with. If there were any more of the Seven Dwarfs around, I was in trouble. Sleepy was bad enough — imagine what Dopey could do.

He wandered out rubbing his eyes, leaving me huddled in a tangled hospital gown and a thickening depression. I had been out of this world for five weeks of Arizona sun, pure desert air and just plain sleeping whole nights through at home. Bliss. But apparently just a detour.

When the radiologist was ushered in by Sleepy, I could hardly believe it. It was Doc to a T. A small, dumpy, twinkly Frenchman, he told me cheerfully, immediately, that his bias was to radiate everything that moved.

"In Europe, in les États-Unis, no question. Untheenkable that you would not go on for radiation therapee. But here in Ontario there ees new thinking. There ees controversy over the usefulness of radiation in some cases."

"This new line comes from Toronto," he added darkly, his contemptuous tone suggesting that Toronto the Good was a cesspool of unhealthy ideas. Degree and kind of treatment depend on the kind and stage of the disease. The norms change as research and studies indicate better approaches, but change comes early or late, depending on where you live. It is a form of geographical roulette.

Until a few years ago, the standard approach to breast cancer was surgery — the Halsted radical mastectomy which includes the major nerves and muscles in the arm and shoulder as well as the breast and often some of the chest wall. If there was no metastasis, then usually there would be no follow-up chemo or radiation. Recently, the thinking has changed; surgeons are no longer quite so quick to remove the whole breast and all around it, if it can be avoided; lumpectomies (the tumour and surrounding tissue) or partial mastectomies (half or more of the breast but with the nipple left intact) are much more common, followed by adjunctive therapy. The extent and kind of therapy are dictated by what stage the cancer is at and how many lymph nodes are infected. (Lymph nodes are removed not in an effort to stop the cancer but as part of the detection procedure: how many nodes infected with cancer cells indicate how far the cancer has spread.) This gentler surgical approach leaves more room for variations in the follow-up treatment. It is in this thicket of choices that patients — and doctors — sometimes get lost.

My case was not clear cut. I hoped Doc was not just making a bad pun when he said this. It was very clearly cut, but whether further treatment after chemo was advisable, was not.

"You will go before the Tumour Board," Doc said.

Tumour Board? Was this something you had to study for? How could there be something with such a straightforward label in this jungle of euphemism? How come it wasn't called Committee of Oncological Research into Malignant Occurrences, for instance? Nope. Tumour Board. Refreshingly blunt. The Board would recommend a course of action and Doc would concur with the majority decision. Medical democracy in action.

Tumour Boards exist in major hospitals all over North America. They are the venue for doctors specializing in various aspects of cancer and cancer therapy to discuss particular cases and offer their opinions on the advantages and disadvantages of alternative treatments.

More waiting — a time during which I plunged right back into the twilight world of cancer. I was sent for another mammogram. Big Deal. What good would that do, given my record with mammograms?

That Other Place

The Tumour Board met on a Thursday: two oncologists, a surgeon, the senior radiologist, Doc and Sleepy. Doc reported that Sleepy had not spoken a word at the meeting, veiling his thoughts from his boss. Like the Dormouse at Alice's tea party, he had probably just nodded off. The two oncologists and the surgeon did not think there was any benefit in radiation treatment for me. Doc disagreed but concurred with the decision for the following reasons: a good deal of time had lapsed since surgery; radiation to the tumour area might prevent recurrence of cancer in that breast but would not prevent a recurrence anywhere else in the body. Since the disease was far more likely to reappear in an organ or the spine, and since there was only about a 15 percent chance of it recurring in the same breast, radiation was not seen to be required.

On the Other Hand. There are so many hands in this country. The Gorgon's head of hands turns you into stone — the inertia of too many choices. On the other hand, Doc said, "Radiation to the tumour site is 100 percent statistically certain to prevent a recurrence in that breast." *Statistically* certain. What was the difference between 100 percent certain and 100 percent *statistically* certain? Of course I didn't ask at the time because I had grabbed the phrase and tucked it into my brain as comfort food for later thought. Finally a certainty. Would I *never* learn?

A statistical certainty is an oxymoron; 100 percent statistically certain means 99 percent certain, that old refrain from the beginning of this journey. In the following months I met several women who were squarely in that one percent statistically impossible category. After radiation to the tumour site, they had a recurrence of cancer in the same place.

The decision was mine. I had been unhooked from the assumption that radiation was unnecessary. Doubts swirled and thickened during the days, and especially the nights, between my first meeting with Sleepy and Doc, and the Board's decision. Did I really have a choice? I had come all this way and now didn't I have to go the extra mile?

Doc was sympathetic and supportive, explaining patiently again and again the ramifications of radiation in my particular case: it would not deter cancer from recurring in any part of my body except the already affected breast. Without it, if the cancer came back in the breast site, the tumour would be harder to detect right away because of all the scar tissue. If it did recur, the next operation would be a full mastectomy, more chemo but no radiation to that part of my body since it would have already received the full dosage allowed.

To sum up: really the main purpose of radiation was to prevent the possible loss of what was left of my breast due to the possible but not probable recurrence of cancer in the same area. How this jibed with the oncologist's pronouncement that I wouldn't survive anyway if there was a recurrence anywhere, I did not know.

But it was one more door to slam on the dragon. Besides, it would only be five more weeks of treatment, albeit this time it would be every day for 25 days except weekends until mid-July. A small price to pay. There was that phrase again. And Doc predicted that side effects would be minimal — sore and cracked skin after a few days of treatment, fatigue probably only toward the end because the radiation target was confined to the breast area, and no body system would be affected.

He even offered me an escape from my own responsibility. Whatever decision I made — to go for treatment or not — and now it really was absolutely up to me; he would agree with and take over as his decision. He had originally offered to make the decision for me, which I could not accept. After all, it was my body and my life. But oddly enough, I found this little skirmish in semantics comforting. I would decide overnight, see him the following morning and he would adopt my decision as his own. I could absolve myself of all responsibility. What difference this would make I don't know. Crazy to be comforted by such a transparent ruse.

It was not an easy decision. Was I opting for further treatment because I didn't want to let go the tangible world of cancer, to abandon the security of a regimen of physical treatment? If I didn't take the radiation treatments, it would mean continuing the journey alone, because instinct told me that I was still very much a traveller.

I was also wary of the "minimal side-effects." After the surprises lurking in the final months of chemotherapy, I viewed with jaundiced eye the assurance that the effects of radiation would be little more than a bad sunburn.

The morning of my appointment with Doc, I walked slowly up the driveway to the clinic, still swithering with indecision, unmindful of the cars and the officious new doorman exercising his bureaucratic powers with the glee of a Third World despot. He stamped and yelled at drivers who lingered too long in discharging their wobbly passengers, he insisted on signed chits from the treatment desk before reluctantly allowing a car to nose into one of the few reserved spots. His predecessor had broken all the rules. He let cars double park, linger in the fire lane, bounce up on the curbs. He had helped patients out of back seats, carrying their shopping bags full of medications, he had unfolded wheelchairs and settled their occupants in the waiting room. He smiled at people, he had time for a word of cheer or a joke.

He didn't last long. His shining human decency was rewarded with a warning to obey the rules or else. He quit and went to work for the Heart Institute ...

As I came slowly and more slowly toward the vortex of the revolving door entrance, out of the sunlight popped the memory of a dream I had had the night before. Its message was so clear I felt as if I were living in the pages of a novel in which the author had resorted to the cheap trick of propelling the plot along with the creaky contrivance of a dream. But this was not fiction.

My dream had been a swirl of mist that transformed into the frothing bubbles in a huge jacuzzi. People were frolicking and playing, the sun shone. A woman stood in the middle of the pool, her back to me. She turned slowly, standing up out of the bubbles, opening her arms wide, her smile empty and sad. Where her right breast should have been was a flat stretch of skin with a gaping slash.

The woman was not me, she was no one I knew, but her expression was one I had seen on so many faces in the clinic, one of terrible resignation.

The Simons Hold a Tumour Board Meeting

I chose to take radiation treatment. To feed another five or six weeks of my life into the cancer hopper would be my last official round in fighting the disease. This time, I wanted it to be a knock-out round. And if it wasn't I would have the wan comfort of knowing that I had done all I could.

-XVI-
The Third Giant Step: Radiation

Radiation [makes tumours shrink or disappear] by damaging the genetic structure (DNA) of the tumor cells so they can't grow or divide ... There is no pain or discomfort during radiation therapy ...

Dollinger *et al.*, Everyone's Guide to Cancer Therapy

It was a different part of the clinic I went to now — the basement, where all the errant radiation beams would be contained. The waiting room was always chock-a-block with people wearing the uniform of the disease, the ubiquitous green gowns with the purple border. We had name tags so that we could wear the same gown each day for the week. One friend flatly refused to wear the standard-issue gown; she said it turned her into a non-person. I didn't really care. It was no more undignified or de-individualizing than what followed after you put the damn thing on.

On my first day, I lay down on the stretcher as directed, full of apprehension. The looming monster of the machine clicked over me as the nurses adjusted the sites. Four people then drew all over me with purple felt pens. Death by paint-by-number.

After defining the target area, measuring and remeasuring, muttering numbers, recalculating them and flicking the lights on and off, they all hustled out of the room leaving me exposed to the glare of the beast. I felt like a sacrifice lying on the altar of cancer; before the blow fell, the high priests had all raced from the church.

The Third Giant Step: Radiation

A sigh from the machine indicated the start of the radiation, another sigh indicated when it was over. Otherwise the machine was silent except for the occasional growl of the compressor. The team scurried back in when the all clear sounded.

"All done," one of them said brightly. "That wasn't so bad, now was it?"

It hadn't hurt, that's true. But the experience lived up to all the apprehension, I am still not sure why. A woman I met at the radiation clinic feared her treatments with an intensity bordering on terror. She agreed that it had nothing to do with physical pain, yet she would be sick every morning before her treatment; she trembled so that the crew would scold her to keep still while the machine did its work. She felt claustrophobic and helpless in its clutches.

"Now, don't get the ink marks wet. See you tomorrow," the head technician said that first day.

"Can't I swim?" I asked in horror. We were in the middle of a typical Ottawa mid-summer heat wave; the temperature hovered in the low 30s with the humidity hitting the 100 percent mark. That entire month of July, with the humidex reading in the mid-40s, people sogged around the city like sponges. And this little bureaucrat was telling me I couldn't swim.

"You mustn't wash off the marks," she said, "We need those to line up the machine each time."

It took me about three days of sweltering at the side of our wonderful, clear, velvety cool lake to realize that the reason I couldn't go in it was because of the inconvenience of losing the target lines, not the danger of being zapped in the wrong place. I swam and swam and watched with perverse satisfaction as the brilliant purple lines faded.

A new team was manning the machine the following day. The team leader clucked in annoyance at the obliterated target but agreed that it was asking a lot to preserve it in its pristine glory through the sweltering heat. Tattoos solved the problem. With a little gun, I was indelibly dotted at the corners of the target area. These spots served as base points from which to redraw the lines every few days for the rest of the treatments. These marks are still there, but ask me if I care. Plunging into the water every evening to wash away the heat and fear and memories of that day's appointment with the monster was worth a whole rash of permanent purple poxes.

My machine was one of the smaller ones — but it was intimidating enough with its battery of jets like eyes, literally boring holes right through you. Something about those treatments baffled me for a long time because in their own way they were almost as bad as chemo. Not physically: chemotherapy simply kicks you in the teeth physically. And many forms of radiation therapy do too. But the kind I had, targeted to a small area where organs were not invaded, was physically not in the same class of hardship as chemo, until the very end.

But psychologically, radiation transforms you from a person — an individual with rights and feelings and emotions — into a slab of poisoned meat. After the technicians drew their indelible target on me, I felt like a carcass with the purple-inked inspection stamp blurred on my flesh.

Like the chemo nurses, the radiology staff were mostly kind, efficient and caring. And well-meaning. One tried to reassure me with an anecdote to prove that even though I was lying there naked from the waist up for the hordes of nurses, students, doctors, the building superintendent, the pizza delivery man, Uncle Tom Cobbler and all to see, no one really saw.

"I wheeled a patient in for treatment to the pelvic area," she said, "and when I came back to ask if she was finished yet, the radiology nurse said, 'What do you mean, she? It's a he.' I hadn't even noticed."

This tale succeeded in making me feel more like a piece of meat than ever. Only now I didn't even know whether I was a ewe or a ram. This feeling intensified when they started to cover my exposed breast with saran wrap. To keep the target forms clean, they said. I just felt microwaved.

On the day of my 22nd treatment, one of the nurses, as she was leaving the room, instructed, "Don't move, now. We don't want to have to redo you." I guess she figured that hunks of brainless flesh that we were, we had to be retrained every day.

The Third Giant Step: Radiation

After 22 treatments, dammit, I knew not to move.

A woman I met later that year, who was undergoing radiation in Saskatoon for breast cancer, had a sweet sort of inadvertent revenge on her crew of nurses. Eileen always carried with her a pair of good luck stones, small, black pebbles, worn smooth with holding. After a treatment one of the stones was missing. Next day she asked the radiology nurses if they had seen it. Had they seen it? They were enraged. The entire clinic had been thrown into turmoil by the magic properties of that innocent little talisman.

Apparently one of them had noticed a small black object on the floor of the treatment room, thought it was cobalt and hit the panic button. No one would touch it. The room was closed off, patients rerouted to other machines. A hardy doctor risked his life by bravely kicking the offending morsel into a container; the nurse, anxious to go off duty, grabbed the canister and ran all the way to the physics department with it, where it was now being analysed by a crew of experts. Eileen wanted it back.

About halfway through my course of radiation, I was shaken by a well-meaning psychologist who told me that cancer specialists, especially radiologists, had no conception of the long-range side effects of radiation.

"They just don't know," he said.

This psychologist spoke of the invasiveness of radiation treatment, that it insulted the body systems (not to mention the dignity and the humanity of the patient) to such an extent that it took from six to eight months for the body to return fully to normal functioning.

I toted up the information I had been given by a variety of people, experts all. One: there would be no side effects from radiation therapy except for mild sunburn. Two: there would be fatigue beginning about halfway through treatment accompanied by severe sunburn. Three: there would be severe sunburn effects, fatigue possibly from day one of treatment which would not really dissipate for a month to six weeks after treatment ended. Four: expect severe skin burn, tight cracked skin, dry mucus glands and tear ducts, sore throat and fatigue lasting for up to eight months.

That Other Place

What was this? I packed my bag to go to Manhattan and in it I put ... Remember that game? A toothbrush. A toothbrush and a comb. A toothbrush, a comb and the entire medicine cabinet. This version was sore skin. Sore skin and fatigue. Sore skin, fatigue, sore throat. Perhaps I could just send the bag and leave myself behind. All this conflicting information was given me by cancer specialists.

By the last treatment my skin was burnt raw and bleeding. My mind was too. My chemo-eyes had come back with a vengeance and I had a permanently sore throat. Doc assured me that the last two symptoms had nothing to do with the treatment. Funny though that the mother of a friend had exactly the same symptoms with the same kind of radiation. A coincidence? Rubbish. Even the small "certainties" now were going down like ninepins. I guess he had forgotten saying to me two months earlier, "There are no experts in cancer, not in the disease or in its treatment. Every patient reacts a different way to both."

But now treatment was over and this time the good feelings did roll in. It had been 13 months from discovery of the lump, through diagnosis of malignancy, confirmation of metastasis and the three giant steps of surgery, chemotherapy and radiation. Physically I was a mess, but I had done everything I could in the way of medical treatment to win Round One — I hoped the only round — with this disease. I had made the decision to go the extra mile, to have radiation, to hurt some more. I had taken some kind of control and it felt good. Now, after such a long journey in this other place, surely I could turn in my passport, leave the night-side of life and return to the kingdom of the well.

-XVII-
Skirmishes on the Medical Front

We should recognize health as a basic right, not a luxury.
Ontario Advisory Council on Women's Issues,
Women and Health, 1988.

In Canada the health care system is founded on the premise that good health is the right of every citizen. Although there has been some skirmishing around the edges of the 'universality' of our social programs, the security net is still in place. Compared to the United States, we have a veritable trampoline of governmental care.

Every time I read or hear about Americans who have backed away from tests and X-rays because of the prohibitive costs, I thank God that I live in Canada because I doubt that I would have gone on with the tracking after the first mammogram indicated that nothing was amiss. My GP's advice to see a surgeon was just that — advice; her words indicated that a second opinion was merely a slightly luxurious precaution more for peace of mind than anything else. Then the surgeon told me exactly the same thing, the old "99 percent certain the lump is benign" line.

This statement is not an uncommon launch into cancer country; Eleanor Bergholz, the journalist who described her bout with cancer in the *New York Times* magazine starts, "It all began routinely enough. When the surgeon examined the lump

That Other Place

in my breast, he was '99 percent certain it's benign.'" When I read that a gong went off in my head. My head reverberated with gongs during the next few months as I read and heard the same thing again and again. It is a consistent detail in the personal accounts of cancer patients I have talked to, accounts I have read, anecdotes I have been told by friends. I was not an aberration of statistics. I was in the mainstream of people whose cancers were diagnosed on the premise that it was 99 percent certain that they did not have cancer.

After the first needle biopsy came back negative, I certainly would have stopped there if faced with a $150 to $200 bill for each additional test or X-ray as is the case in the States.

Allen had a boating accident in Arizona that landed him in hospital in that state for a few days of breath-taking costs: he was billed $1.65 for a doll's-sized tube of toothpaste approximately enough for one tooth; each demerol injection set him back $10.95; each X-ray, and there were many, cost $135.00; I think they were trying to find his wallet. Room-service X-rays, when the technician wheeled in an enormous machine to zap him in situ cost twice as much. The ticking we heard as the machine rolled sonorously through the door, I realize now, must have been the dollar meter.

Lucky for us the hospital was not charging by the foot for the length of tube that had to be inserted through the chest wall into Allen's lung. The cost of his room, a lovely sun-lit private space, was astronomical, and did not include medical care, just the bed, maybe the pillows. The care was excellent and gold-plated. The doctors were superb and platinum. Without Canadian coverage we'd have had to sell the farm.

Here in Ontario, OHIP allows you some degree of financial equanimity in the event of hospitalization and out-patient treatment. You can be relatively thoughtless about pursuing tests which have a "99 percent certainty" of finding nothing. Of course there is abuse of the system — doctors whipping their patients through at the rate of knots to build up their billings; people going to the doctor again and again for non-existent conditions or for a sore throat or cold that would clear up in a day or two anyway. But these abuses are worth it, if the system provides accessible universal health care that saves lives and eases pain.

So indeed, we should all look upon good health as a right. But once you lose it, it becomes a luxury simply because you can't demand it back. You can't go to court and sue for the return of your health. You must fight for its return. Our health system is an ally in the fight, but there is a lot that you, as patient, can do to help.

All the literature on alternative treatments to cancer — treatments that are not in the medical mainstream — emphasize the importance of taking control. Don't be a "patient" waiting passively for things to be done to you by doctors; be a partner with your doctor, be the leader, the ultimate decision-maker. Although being an abject follower is tempting because if things don't work out you always have someone else to blame. "That dumb doctor, what does he know, him and his stupid treatment, and now just look at me." Of course, this perverse satisfaction is hard to enjoy if you are dead.

At the beginning, I was utterly intimidated by the Simons of my new world, the medical experts, the Authorities. First of all, they get to stand up, while you get to lie down, usually in an undignified position. Then they talk over your head with each other as if you are stone deaf. They don't like it when you tug their sleeves and say, "Hey, hey what about me?" in a small voice. But do it anyway. It will make you feel better, and that's what it's all about, yes?

They get to wear clothes when you don't. You get to cower inside a flimsy little gown that gapes either front or back, depending on how you put it on. Even that was a decision I had trouble making. At first, I actually worried about the right way to wear the gown. I remember one utterly pathetic moment as I stood in the cubicle studying intently the instructions on the wall on how to wear the damn thing. It was important to put it on the right way, to follow all the rules. Did I really care? Did anyone care? Did I care if anyone cared? It appears that I did, in the beginning.

That Other Place

Clutching the gown around me, trailing ties, I crept out to sit in the waiting room, only to be herded back by an officious nurse: "Wait in the cubicle until your name is called," she ordered brusquely, flapping her clipboard at me. And I meekly did as bidden. I did not ask why, I just sat on the little bench, the walls closing in on either side, wondering idly if this was necessary. But I stayed there.

Was this miserable little wimp really me? No, it was another person who entered my body with the cancer. Eventually I ousted her, though. When I realized that she had taken up residence, snivelling creature that she was, I spent hours planning her eviction. She disappeared slowly over the next few months as the fear subsided to a manageable level. A few months later, at the same clinic, for the same tests, the same nurse said the same thing to me. I fixed her with a steely glare and continued on my way to the waiting room. It seems hard to believe now that such a tiny victory gave me such an inordinate burst of satisfaction.

Shortly after this I won an even greater battle, but it was an easier fight because it was for Sam and not for myself.

He had gone skiing with friends. The phone rang mid-morning: "Mrs. Williams? This is the ski patrol at Camp Fortune calling."

Oh God.

"Your son has had a bad fall. He's fine, just winded himself but he doesn't want to ski any more today."

Camp Fortune is about 25 minutes from Ottawa. I got there that morning in about two, all the way trying to guess what the ski patroller hadn't told me. The first-aid room of a ski area does not phone to say your kid is tired and doesn't feel like skiing any more.

The hidden message grew clear when I saw Sam. Doubled over with pain, he could hardly get into the car. His freckles stood out against the pallor of his face; despite the biting cold, perspiration lay on his forehead. The caller was a master of understatement. Indeed, Sam didn't want to ski any more that day. How about that winter?

Skirmishes on the Medical Front

A time-series of X-rays at the emergency department of the hospital established the problem. Kidney damage. He was now vomiting every few minutes from the pain; Allen and Matt arrived and we all sat close to Sam, who lay on a stretcher waiting for the ambulance to take him and me to the children's hospital.

We waited, not talking a lot, willing the pain to abate. A small mean nurse snicked up to us, "Only two visitors to a patient," she snapped. "And those chairs are for patients, not for visitors. You'll have to stand."

We were in a hallway, for godsake. There wasn't a soul in sight, just our tight worried little group. The only "patient" was a 14-year-old kid who couldn't have sat in a chair if his life depended on it, who could have no relief in painkillers until the extent of the damage was established, who was scared, who hurt, and whose only comfort was his family. And this paragon of bureaucracy was trying to chase us away with a spout full of rules.

Before Allen could chew her into small pieces, I snarled a line or two, the message of which was clear: Listen, you jerk. This is my son. We are all staying right here with him. We are sitting down to do so. Take a hike.

She did.

Most kids, if they have to break anything in a ski accident, break an ankle, a leg, maybe a collar bone. Not Sam. He had broken his kidney. Split it right across. The next two weeks he spent in the children's hospital, bed-bound and bored ... with nothing but the best of care.

Two months later, Matt came to grief on the rugby field; he phoned in a wavering voice to say that he had had a bit of an accident, nothing to worry about, but could I come and fetch him and the car because his coach would not allow him to drive home.

Déjà vu. I arrived to find him stretched out on the grass verge, like a civil war leftover, his head bound in a bloodied rag, his nose squashed sideways, one eye swollen shut, a gash through his eyebrow, and an ankle the size of a melon. Off to the emergency department again. Enough already. I honed my tongue in readiness for the snippy nurse, but she didn't break cover. A wonderful young doctor sewed up Matt's head, X-rayed his broken nose and sent him home on crutches. She gave him a handful of painkillers and a lot of sympathy. I wanted to apologize to her for all my bad feelings about some of her colleagues. The next day when another, equally sympathetic, doctor set Matt's nose, dragging it back from what seemed to be about the middle of his cheek, it was me and not Matt who whimpered and swayed.

Between Sam's kidney and Matt's nose was Allen's neck. He'd had X-rays at Christmas because of persistent pain in his shoulders and neck, and numbness in his hands. At the time he had been told that his X-rays showed nothing abnormal. Three months later, someone in radiology apparently got around to looking at the film close up and phoned to say that in fact there was a problem. Did this make sense? Not at all. Why was he told three months earlier that all was fine if no one had checked the X-rays? Medicine moves in mysterious ways.

"There is a shadow on the vertebrae in your neck. We want you to have a CAT scan," he was told by his doctor, presumably a blind one, since it had been he who originally had given the all-clear.

What could it be, this shadow? The answer was bafflegab. Not once was the word "cancer" mentioned, but it may as well have been spelled out in nine-foot neon letters on the doctor's forehead. An appointment was made for the scan ... for a month later.

When Allen told me, I went to pieces. I railed, I ranted, I cried and thumped walls.

"Tell them you have a wife with cancer who is going to go right around the twist if we have to wait a month with this hanging over our heads. I CAN'T STAND IT!" This was not a cancer personality talking. This was a banshee. The Capricorn line had been crossed and I was on the rampage.

Allen had the scan three days later, Sunday night at 10 p.m. The hasty rebooking was the work of a very humane radiologist, who also phoned within two days to say that the shadow was on the film and not on Allen's neck. All was OK.

The hospital wards are not seething with monsters, but sometimes in this journey it seemed like it. It's the 99 percent syndrome again: 99 percent are good, caring, benign. It's the one percent that get your attention.

-XVIII-
Doctor as God

> Algernon: The doctor's found out that Bunbury could not live, that is what I mean — so Bunbury died.
> Lady Bracknell: He seems to have had great confidence in the opinion of his physicians ...
>
> Oscar Wilde, *The Importance of Being Earnest*

In the year of diagnosis, surgery, chemo and radiation, and the years since of check-ups, tests and tracking, I have met a variety of doctors, nurses, clinicians and attitudes. I have heard myriad stories about the good, the bad and the downright terrifying who rule cancer clinics and waiting rooms. I have read reams, seen films and videos and interviewed medical people throughout Canada. Sometimes I feel like a foreign correspondent, reporting on a war taking place somewhere else. Occasionally I surface in the thick of the fray.

At first I didn't take sides: doctors said "do this" and who was I to quibble? When the surgeon said that he would operate as soon as possible after diagnosis was confirmed, did I argue? Are you kidding? He was the expert, he was God, and I never thought of questioning him. In the midst of the panic and fear, my reeling instincts agreed with him anyway. But I wonder now, if he had said, "We have to cut off your head," would I have been so malleable? Probably, nodding dumbly in agreement while I still had a head to nod with.

When the oncologist prescribed aggressive chemotherapy, I concurred, a concurrence that was slightly more considered on my part, but I was still pretty much on automatic pilot on this new route. Even though I wasn't questioning yet, I found myself blaming the doctors for my presence in this new country at all and stumbled into the front line with all the other walking wounded, complaining that, on the whole, doctors were brutal/evasive/bland/stupid/cruel and egregious liars.

My journey was peppered with doctors and nurses whose throats I would have cheerfully throttled. These were the ones who demanded obedience to such meaningless bureaucratic procedures as the requirement for patients to change into pyjamas or nightgowns on admittance to hospital for surgery even though absolutely nothing was going to happen until the next day; or the ones who insisted on having people wait inside the cubicles for changing clothes until their turn came for blood tests, X-rays, whatever; or the hospital emergency staff who refused to allow a mother in to her injured daughter because she was 18 years old, an adult who presumably needed no comfort after being savaged by a dog (ours, as it happens, but that's another story). Perhaps these instances are trivial in the overall scheme of things — but each one could be the last straw in a traumatic experience made worse by the thoughtless and dehumanizing treatment of the very people you trust will help you.

And then there are the not so trivial actions, such as the refusal of an officious little nurse to administer a painkiller more often than every four hours — "He could develop an addiction!" to an 89-year-old dying patient. And how else can you react but with fury when you remember that doctor who told his patient that yes, her tests indicated that she had a brain tumour but no, nothing could be done until it had grown from stage one to stage three or four. Come back and see me then, he said. And this was over the phone. Perhaps this approach is understandable from a strictly medical viewpoint. It is unforgivable from a humanitarian viewpoint.

In such cases, shooting the messenger is the only answer. Maybe this doctor was such a sensitive little flower, he couldn't deliver the news face to face. If so, then he shouldn't be an oncologist. Or perhaps this was his way of dealing with burnout — shielding himself from the blistering heat of the pain and fear of his patient who had just, as far as she was concerned, received a death warrant — in order to continue practising. Or maybe, to give him the benefit of the doubt, he was already burned out, but unfortunately still smouldering.

Doctors who deal with cancer as if it were under a microscope in a lab rather than spreading its malignant force through a person's body skewer their patients on scientific facts unblunted by sympathy or hope.

Of course, doctors have to make excruciatingly tough decisions about patients, their chances, the right treatment, protocol and dosages. They live in a forest of judgement calls. Some make decisions better than others. Some convey those decisions better than others.

The oncologist of a friend was one who should have kept his mouth shut and left the conveying to others. Janine had just talked to her oncologist when I met her in the waiting room of the cancer clinic. And apparently, he had just talked to God, because he had slammed the door on all hope. The doctor had, not God.

Janine's cancer had spread to her lungs, her liver, her thyroid. You name it. Five minutes before I saw her, she had been told, No, there was nothing more to be done. Go home now.

"But what about this new drug, Janine?" I asked, me, who knew all about the pitfalls of the popular press announcements of new cancer cures. I should have known better. "It has been approved for use in Canada. Can't you get that?"

"I asked about it. I am being punished apparently," she said with a snap of rage. "Because I've had two cancers, and because I have had cysplatin [a particularly strong chemotherapy drug], they won't give it to me."

"Why not? Why not, if it might help?"

"There is so little of the drug, it comes from the bark of a tree that grows only on high hillsides or something," she waved her hand dismissively. "I am a bad risk. I might be bad for their statistics."

She had already defied statistics by surviving three and a half years with stage 3/4 ovarian cancer. Six months before that she had breast cancer, apparently unrelated. That was a mistake.

Not the diagnosis, but having two versions of cancer. This provided a bureaucratic loophole for the doctor to dive through in support of his decision. He told her that it was just possible that her recurrences of cancer stemmed from the breast cancer, not the ovarian, and since they didn't know for sure, they wouldn't chance using the new drug. It was so scarce they would have to preserve it for "more certain outcomes."

Until that day, there had never been a question as to which of her two cancers was recurring. It was the ovarian cancer that was on the rampage; the apparently completely unrelated breast cancer had disappeared with the first wave of chemotherapy.

"I asked Dr. X, 'If I was the Prime Minister's wife, would you give me the new drug.' 'Yes, he said, But only for comfort.'"

Comfort? Whose? The nation's? This sounded like a cold political comfort to me. Certainly there was no crumb for Janine. She was waiting to see another oncologist, to ask for help in bolstering her immune system so that she could continue the fight on her own. She was given no help, either in the form of physical treatment or psychological support.

At this point I was called in for my examination. A complete stranger swept into the room, sat down and asked in a friendly manner, "How are you ... uh ... Madame Williams?" consulting the file in his hand.

"Fine, thank you, how are you ... uh ...?" I paused, having no file to consult.

"Fine, too." He looked at me expectantly. I looked back. Silence. Finally I spoke. "Well, now I know how you are, but I don't know who you are."

He was surprised. "But I am the senior specialist for gynaecology, Dr. X."

"How do you do, Dr. X. But why am I seeing you? I thought this was a breast cancer check-up."

"Ah, no, Dr. Y asked me to see you."

He did not explain why, and I was sufficiently unhinged by my conversation with Janine five minutes before that I did not ask. We started over again.

"Now, how are you?" he asked a second time.
I was still fine.
"*Bien*. So no worries. Until next time, then." He jumped to his feet.
"That's all?"
"*Oui*, that's all." He smiled a charming smile.
"Well, no wait. Since I am here, I'd like to ask you about something."
He sat down again.
"I read about a blood test that can detect ovarian cancer. I wonder if I could have that test since that seems to be why I am seeing you rather than Dr. Y. I mean you are a gynaecologist and I had mentioned some symptoms that seemed unrelated to breast but could be ..." I tailed off.
"Where did you read about this test?"
"Uh, *Peop*le magazine," I said somewhat shamefaced at having to admit my less than impeccable medical source. "There was an article about Gene Wilder who gave evidence before an American House Committee. He claimed, and had several oncologists' support, that if his wife, Gilda Radner, had been given this test early on, her ovarian cancer would have been detected sooner and she'd have had a much better chance at beating the disease, at least for a while."

The doctor's eyes blinked with boredom as I spoke. I guessed that since that issue of *People* magazine was published a couple of weeks earlier, he had been asked the question dozens of times. His reply was seamless.

"That blood test is CA 125. It is entirely inconclusive. It can show positive results with benign problems, it can produce negative results in a woman with obvious disease."
"So it is not a good idea?"
"Non. It can be very misleading. Besides, you should not be concerned, you do not have ovarian cancer yet." He smiled again and left.
"Excuse me? Did you say 'yet'?" I whispered to the empty room. This was another doctor who shouldn't be allowed to open his mouth. Surely I had misheard? I did not have ovarian

cancer ... yet? That is exactly what he said. Verbatim. Perhaps it was an idiosyncrasy of language, since English was not his mother tongue. But that kind of reassurance sounds no better in French. For such a sensitive doctor he'd make a fine mortician.

That very same day, the *Ottawa Citizen* carried a story about the new drug, called taxol, about which Janine had asked. It is made from the bark of a rare yew tree that grows only sparsely in the Pacific Northwest. It takes six 100-year-old Pacific yews to treat one patient, according to the article. Studies are showing that it is particularly effective in the treatment of advanced ovarian and breast cancer (such as Janine's).

Dr. Samuel Brodes, director of the National Cancer Institute in Bethesda, Maryland, is quoted as saying "[It is] the most important new drug we have had in cancer for 15 years. I'm not saying it's a cure, but I will tell you there are women who failed every other treatment who responded." Interesting semantics in Dr. Brodes' statement. It is not the treatment that failed the women, but the women who failed the treatment ... Apparently it is not found in the United States. The Canadian government, in its wisdom, is exporting the bark to the United States, making the drug even harder to get in Canada.

The irony of it all made me weep. Yes, we have a drug. Yes, it is proving to be almost miraculous. But no, you can't have it, Janine. Why not? Oh, because you are a bad statistical risk and besides, there isn't enough to treat everybody, especially since we are busily shipping it out of the country. In less than two months, Janine was dead. Hope had been withdrawn.

There are also the doctors who deal with patients in exactly the opposite way, trying to soften their truths by hiding in a thicket of medicalese and hazy platitudes. "Doctors are particularly likely to pull the wool over your eyes in relation to cancer. This is partly because they themselves find it difficult to cope with the emotional intensity of clear statements. It is partly because they need to believe in unrealistic expectations in order to keep the entire cancer-treatment machine rumbling along." (Fulder, p.118)

That Other Place

The "entire cancer treatment machine" rumbles along on faith, for which thank God, and on creaky wheels oiled by statistics. It is the only foundation upon which research can stand. But statistics are wily little chameleons, showing a different face at every turn. They are especially vicious in the mouths of doctors on a one-to-one basis with a newly diagnosed, bewildered, desperate cancer patient. It is a no-win situation for both players.

The doctor can speak with certainty only about the statistical history of the disease; and these statistics, at least in relation to breast cancer, reveal a debilitating stasis in the treatment-success rate. According to one source, 60 to 80 percent of breast cancer patients will survive for five years (depending on who's keeping track) but only 10 percent will escape their cancer altogether. (I guess this means that they will die of something else entirely, not that they will live forever.) This same harbinger of joy claims that "[t]his is probably no more than the real cure rate of 100 years ago." (Fulder, p. 116)

But the patient isn't a statistic. Right away, what we have here is a breakdown in communication. The gulf widens as the doctor, as my oncologist did, stays on the stats side of the widening gulf, and the patient, as I did, tries to shake away the mists of misery to clutch onto the most important fact of all, and one that statistics cloud unmercifully. You are not a statistic, you are not a disease, you are an individual, with an individual set of responses, emotions and immune systems, and therefore you have as much chance as anyone in the world to be the one that gets better. And statistics, like piranha fish, keep tearing away at that belief.

But what else can the doctor do? Many lie in an even more blatant way than statistics do, with the best intentions. By either downplaying the stage of the cancer, or whisking away all hope by pronouncing that treatment can do nothing more, they weaken the patient's motive to fight the disease. They are often reluctant to provide anything but the barest bones of information, thus pushing the patients to the sidelines of their own battle.

Doctor as God

In Japan they go even further. Apparently there is such shame associated with cancer that eight out of ten doctors in that country lie to their patients. They say that the cancer is a stomach ulcer, an ovarian cyst, anything but the truth. When the Emperor Hirohito was dying of cancer, the palace spokesman never once mentioned the disease by name, and the newspapers did not report it as cancer until the editors were assured that the Emperor was too weak to read the papers.

This attitude casts doubt on the oft-quoted statistics claiming that the incidence of breast cancer among Japanese women is 50 percent lower than in women in North America. Perhaps it is just in the reporting — like suicide rates in Ireland or other predominantly Catholic countries where death by suicide is hushed up and reported usually as death by accident.

In Simone de Beauvoir's moving account of her mother's death, she wrestles with the guilt of lying to her mother, encouraging her to believe that she had been operated on for peritonitis, not cancer. It was a combined decision — of the doctors as well as de Beauvoir and her sister — to keep the truth from her mother. The deception added an excruciating layer to the already painful process of facing her mother's dying. And it removed any control or power her mother might have had in being allowed to face the truth.

My father died of cancer. Emergency surgery confirmed the spread of the disease; there was nothing to be done. There was no question of lying to him. He had the right to know. To deny him the truth would have been to deny him as an individual.

His surgeon was a fine, sensitive man, who had been willing to risk major surgery in the hope of fixing the problem, when most practitioners would not have bothered with a patient of 89 years. He took my brothers and me to the recovery room at midnight to see Dad; the nurse there was irritated and tried to refuse us entry — the rules said no visitors in the recovery room, no matter what the circumstances. The surgeon quietly pulled rank. We were gowned and masked, and allowed in.

The afternoon after Dad's operation, when I came to his room, I met a covey of doctors on their rounds. "Has Dr. S. told my father that it is cancer?" I asked.

The head doctor frowned in exasperation. "Of course not. Your father is in no condition to be told that. A man of his advanced age? He is far too confused with the anaesthetic. Dr. S. won't be telling him for a while."

I waited while they swept in around Dad's bed. One of them bent over him and shouted, "And how are we today, Mr. F.?" I so much wanted Dad to answer, "I don't know how you feel, you dimwit, but I feel lousy."

He didn't. What he did say had as much effect though. "Not so good," he said quietly. "But as I suspected, Dr. S. says it's cancer."

I have such a powerful image of the four doctors, their heads lifting in unison, like startled deer in a clearing, swivelling their round, nervous eyes at me where I stood in the doorway. They had been caught out in their superior, smug "We're-the-experts" reply to me. Part of their surprise was the reminder that this patient was a person, not a disease, not a statistic, not a helpless old man to be condescended to, but a strong individual with rights, and faculties and an intelligence that far exceeded all theirs put together. He was my father and he had put them to rout.

Perhaps it is the very nature and reputation of the disease that unmans the medical profession. Renate Rubinstein writes that before she got multiple sclerosis she had taken for granted that in our age a good doctor can cure anything, "as long as it isn't cancer." (p. 25)

Mostly, I have more sympathy with doctors now than I did earlier on this journey. Patients' expectations are so encompassing — some expect doctors to be God, to make it better, and if they don't, they, and not the disease, get the blame. Others want the doctor to tell them only what they want to hear. Even if the doctor doesn't do that, some patients' powers of selective hearing allow them to hear it anyway. As Rubinstein says, "Self-deceit comes naturally."

Just at the end of my radiation treatment, I received a phone call from a friend of a friend. Her voice was strong and the tremors barely discernible. "I have just found out that I have breast cancer," she said as if she had just discovered that she had a food allergy. The apparent confidence in her tone did not hide the fear. "What happens now?"

I was tongue-tied. I wanted desperately to reassure her, to say, hey listen, it's tough for a while, but you'll get through it. You have six lymph nodes affected? No problem, the chemo will take care of that. And in a year you'll be laughing.

That's what doctors probably want to say too, but they can't. It might happen that way, but they must hedge their bets. I could hear my voice growing as hearty as the caller's, but all I could offer in comfort was, not statistics, God forbid, but my own experience, not because it was so great but because we had a lot in common. There is comfort in knowing that you are not alone on this journey.

One of my solutions for dealing with dispatches from the medical world was to filter them through the doctor in the family. My niece, Nicole, continually helped me through the medical thickets — putting out the brush fires of fear with explanations and facts. After each foray into the oncologist's office those first few months, where I feverishly wrote everything down and still got half of it wrong, I would depend on her to translate it all into words of one syllable that even my panicked brain could grasp. However, not even Nicole could translate one beaut of a consultation, the first tracking session I had after radiation treatments were finished.

The clinic was full to bursting — people in various states of disrepair lined the hallways, their faces awash with decrepitude and hope. I had to keep swallowing and swallowing to keep the sudden welling of nausea under control, even before I got into the clinic. Walking along the outside of the building with eyes averted from the chemo room windows, slowing to a snail's pace as I went through the revolving doors, I wanted to turn and bolt. Despite the kindness of the staff, God how I hated the place.

Downstairs for "blood work." Bloody work. I sat and waited for a little while, watching a nurse with her back to me, working at a machine. I remembered what the Vancouver hospital administrator had said about cancer patients — "cancer patients like to wait" so I asked brightly if there was someone coming to take my blood soon.

She turned slowly and deliberately on her stool, fixed me with a gimlet eye and said, spacing her words evenly, "Sit down please and wait."

I backed up and sat down obediently, not even a whimper of protest while she fiddled and messed about with a microscope. The symbolism was perfect: I, a human being, was second in line to a cell or two on a glass slide.

A few minutes later, back up in the examination room, a doctor swept in, not one I had ever seen before. He may have been a relation of The Brain though, there was something in his speech patterns ... Except his name was many syllables longer. It sounded rather like Wyzinklavinskyatski. He was gentle in his examination and gave me no bad news. He gave me no good news. He gave me no news at all. Or maybe he gave me all sorts of news, but I could understand perhaps one word in a hundred. I think he told me that his son had had chemotherapy, or maybe an appendectomy. Why he would have told me about either I don't know, since we were discussing radiation. At least I think we were.

Just before leaving, he said "Meesus Villmns. This paper take to the place where you are passing every day. All is quiet. Stay in the stable now."

He shook my hand with fervour and backed out of the room. Perhaps he wasn't a doctor at all. Maybe he was a vet?

The relationship between doctor and patient is crucial, and worth working at. If your relations are confrontational, if there is no trust, then you are up against a double enemy. You have the disease to fight as well as the frustration and anger created by bad connections with your doctor. Best to try and find another. This is easy advice to give, you will find it in all the literature, but often it is difficult to follow. It takes courage to up and tell a doctor — The Authority — that you would prefer someone else, thanks, and please could you have your medical records?

Doctor as God

In some instances, doctors refuse to provide those records, claiming that they are the property of his or her office or clinic. Wrong. They are yours, and you are absolutely within your rights to take, or have them sent, to another doctor.

Part way through this journey I started to gain back control of my own reactions — I was chagrined to find myself riding other people's wave of anger and cynicism. Maybe it has been just luck, but the main doctors who have guided the various stages of my medical treatment have been the best: my GP whose instinct told her that not all was right, despite test results to the contrary; a surgeon with magic hands and a heart that tried to encompass all the pain; an oncologist whose straight talk and intelligent, sympathetic care helped steady me on a shaky course; a radiologist who responded to psychological needs far beyond the boundaries of the physical treatment, and especially Nicole, my personal guide through the medical maze.

I have also encountered some Bad Eggs — egotistical, fanatical, monumentally insensitive creatures, but they have been peripheral players on my journey. These brief encounters with such Simons and the experiences of those all around me indicate the crucial importance of good doctors. It's worth the effort, the stress, the possible confrontation, to find them because they are there. In fact, even in the last five years, there has been a shift in the curricula of medical schools toward the human element in a doctor's training. Another ray of hope in this other place where each of us will travel at some time or another.

June 1990
I visited Sylvia in hospital on Friday; she has a partial blockage of the colon — "inflammation" she said. She looked beautiful, her eyes large and knowing. "I know what they are telling me," she said. "I don't think I am in denial."

-XIX-
On and Off the Bandwagons

There is no sign that impostors, charlatans, and the plain misguided have diminished in numbers since the Middle Ages.

Philip Ward, Preface, *Common Fallacies* II

After you get run over by the truck that is cancer and you stagger back to your feet wondering what hit you, along come the bandwagons. They roar down on you like gangbusters, and you dodge and hop out of their path, at the same time trying to balance a perspective that has been splintered every which way but loose.

You have now entered the freeways of Lunatic Therapy, a whole new world of spaghetti junctions, forks in the road and cul de sacs. Unfortunately this area has been lumped in with all alternative therapies by most conventional practitioners, a blinkered attitude that is often as limiting and destructive as the therapy it condemns.

So you, as the patient, must become your own doctor in a sense, straining all the theories through stable, balanced analysis and good judgement, both which of course have been knocked senseless. Never mind that your brain is incapable of choosing anything more important than which TV program to veg out on; despite the seemingly terminal paralysis of fear and desperation, you must be selective. Many of the wagons will just take you on a mystery tour that ends nowhere. But don't let them all roll by without at least checking them out, because among the exhaust fumes and dust there might be one that will really help.

Of course, they are not restricted to cancer country, these vehicles of promise. From the garages of religion, language, politics, social attitudes, they roll, their drivers insisting on the most bizarre of currency as the price of a boarding ticket.

Take language fads: we are no longer supposed to use the term "handicapped" to describe people with conditions that handicap them. For a while we were allowed to say "disabled persons" (not "the disabled") but now "challenged people" is decreed as the accepted term ... that's this year. "Physically challenged," "mentally challenged," how about "ridiculously challenged." Even a reissue of the movie version of Grimm's classic tale of Snow White scrambled to be politically correct. To their credit, the distributors did not rename the film *Snow White and the Seven Height Challenged Persons,* but they came up with the next best solution. They seemed to have dropped the Dwarfs right off the marquee. There was nothing they could do to clean up Dopey's act though. He's still the archetypical village idiot, pure and SIMPLE — no amount of 1990s hindsight sanitization could remedy old Dopey, thank goodness.

Feminist thinking founders on the extremities of language sensitivities. The most recent linguistic straitjacket? The term "single" parent is being ousted by "lone" parent. "Single" apparently has the connotation of unmarried status so is verboten. "Lone" brings Hop-Along Cassidy to my mind, but to each his (l)own ... And "female," for some inexplicable reason has been pushed aside by "woman" even as an adjective, as in "women trends," a fine illustration of the growing insanity of language bent all out of shape in an attempt to be politically correct.

Oddly enough, in the area of disease and language, the trend is drifting the opposite direction. It used to be that cancer was a shameful affliction, unlike heart disease, which still enjoys a much higher social acceptance. Thus, no one ever had "cancer" right out loud. But now, at least in North America, there seems to be a move in the direction of calling a spade a spade, or a tumour a tumour.

On and Off the Bandwagons

I thought I was one of those "cancerites" in the language vanguard, avoiding euphemisms in favour of the cold hard currency of realism. It came as an unpleasant shock when, despite all my brave words, I found myself not in the lead waving a flag saying CANCER, but trailing the parade, hoping no cameras would pick me out of the crowd. At my first meeting of a self-help group for cancer patients, I almost pretended to be going somewhere else when I spotted the shamelessly posted notice on the bulletin board: "Cancer Meeting, School Library, 7:30." The only difference between Hester Prynne and me was that my scarlet letter was C. I wanted to slink in under a euphemism. Either that or wear a bag over my head. But those were early days yet, and all sorts of attitudes later fell by the wayside.

Jacquelyn Johnson, author of *Intimacy: Living as a Woman after Cancer,* makes a good point (among many): she never uses the term "cancer patient" except in a quotation. She writes, "In this book, you will not see the word patient except in this sentence and when quoted directly. We are women who have or who had cancer, not patients or cancer cases." (p. 31)

Language is a powerful influence, overt as well as covert. The term "cancer patient" suggests a passivity we could all do without, conjuring up images of the waiting rooms at the cancer clinic, where patience is almost palpable. Rumour has it that the heart clinic waiting rooms are filled with impatients — blustery individuals who expect, demand and get.

But what is a catchy alternative? "Cancerites" won't do. What about "cancerously challenged persons"? Uh. No. "People who have or have had cancer" falls into the same category as "Persons with disabilities" — mealy mouthfuls of porridge words.

Bernie Siegel calls people who fight their cancer "Exceptional Patients," because they are willing to take responsibility and participate in the struggle against their illness by looking at their lives, seeing how they might change. He calls such people "respants" — responsible participants. Weeell, I think maybe I'd rather be a victor, which is Benjamin's term, than a respant, which conjures up images of old Zekie, a cairn terrier from my

That Other Place

childhood, who spent his summers lying panting in the cool earth under the lilac. Benjamin defines "victor" as "a person who has been diagnosed as having cancer and has taken back some control in his life, has become a Patient Active, and considers himself a Victor, no matter what his physical condition." (Introduction) My only quibble with his definition is its exclusion of female victor ... I mean "woman" victors.

Death is still shrouded in mysterious, distancing terms. People don't die, they pass away. Motors are allowed to die; so is laughter and the wind; but people go to their last home or their final reward; sometimes, in fits of irreverence or hysteria, they check out or bite the dust, expressions that still attempt to keep death at bay.

Religion has spewed forth the granddaddies of bandwagons since the beginning of human thought. They careen out of the mainstream, spinning their wheels in an attempt to mow each other down. Road-sharing is a totally foreign concept. Science certainly has its share; the flat-earthers drove their wagons in tight circles for fear of falling off the edge: the round-earthers bravely drove into the horizon and didn't fall off, at which point their vehicles disappeared into the maw of fact.

These days, one of the busiest roads is the one of "personal growth." Theories, exercises, therapies, treatises abound. Some are new and fascinating, some restate the obvious in a new cloak of semantics; some clank along shedding bits of logic; some are just plain nuts, and some are dangerous.

The New Age throngs with such routes to self-awareness and improvement as energy balancing, channelling, reflexology, rolfing, soul travel, sound and light healing, metamorphic technique, rebirthing, astro-synthesis, gestalt, reiki, trager, acupuncture, shinjin, Alexander technique, art therapy, crystal work, therapeutic touch, subud, yoga — the list goes on. In Ottawa, a city not noted for its whimsy, there are organizations such as Inner Peace Unlimited, Canadian College of Kineseography, Church of Perfect Liberty, Institute for Planetary Evolution, Movements of Spiritual Inner Awareness Canada ... No question, it is a growth industry to rival robotics.

On and Off the Bandwagons

These movements are not restricted to North America, nor are they unique to our times. It seems every generation has its "New Age" fringe activities. In 1922, Katherine Mansfield, the New Zealand writer who suffered from tuberculosis, was persuaded by A.R Orage, the editor of a weekly entitled *New Age*, to put herself in the hands of the Russian mystic healer, Gurdjieff. She had tried every route to recovery and "the miracle never came near happening." Orage had given her a copy of a book entitled *Cosmic Anatomy*, which fascinated her, but it was unlikely that Katherine, or anybody else, understood the "book's peculiar combination of theosophy, Hinduism, astrology, cryptic diagrams, pseudo-physics and false etymology .... [couched in a] pretentious mixture of tortuous language and muddled thought ... dogmatism and contradictions." (Meyers, p. 239) This description applies to many of the titles thronging the shelves of New Age bookshops today. The book helped convince Katherine, in a last desperate bid for recovery, to go to Gurdjieff's institute in France, a decision that probably hastened her death.

Gurdjieff taught that the "harmonious integration of the physical, emotional and mental centres of man could be achieved by a method of conscious effort and voluntary suffering." (*Ibid.*, p. 246) Scarcely able to walk or breathe ("My cough is so much worse that I *am* a cough — a living, walking or lying-down cough" (*Ibid.*, p. 243), Katherine spent that last six weeks of her life on a platform over a cow stable inhaling the fetid stench of the animals. This was to "renew her strength through the radiation of animal magnetism ..." (*Ibid.,* p. 250) She died on that platform, amongst the fumes of manure and the mad fanaticism of her "healer." She was 34.

When you are lurking around rock bottom both mentally and physically, brought there by illness, grief, depression, loss, whatever it might be, that's when the bandwagons rolling past the grimy cellar window look the most appealing. And that is when you must be most wary. The toughest task is to sort out the ones that might take you somewhere other than a balcony over a cowshed.

That Other Place

The byways of cancer are particularly busy with them, steaming along scooping up the willing, the eager, the naive, the desperate. People positively leap from the hedgerows, scrambling to board the vehicle of dreams with their banners proclaiming the latest and fashionable orthodoxies of the day.

After diagnosis, surgery and the early days of chemo came a time when I was most vulnerable. A line kept wafting through my brain — a book title, *So Far Down It Looks Like Up to Me*. Well, there is a sub-basement so much further down there is no up. It was from there that I found myself trying to jump on every bandwagon I could find. I didn't even wait for them to come down my street. Luckily though, I didn't have the energy to do much more than read about them and long for the instant miracles they promised.

One area in which my lack of energy and self-discipline kept me from going haywire was diet. Let me hasten to say nutrition is not a bandwagon; good nutrition is a wise and proven vehicle to good health. But some of the spin-offs are exceeding weird. Mark Twain wisely warned: "Be careful of reading health books. You may die of a misprint." There are also health books that could hasten the end without any help from misprints. Among its horrific instructions on how to achieve the good life, one such book exhorted its readers to drink lots of liquid salad; this nutritional delicacy you were to make yourself every morning instead of coffee: throw lettuce in a blender, grind it to mush, add nothing — no salt, no pepper, not even a healthy dollop of mayonnaise — and drink it. Several times a day. The author claims that this, among other noxious tortures, had kept her healthy for eight years after her bout with cancer. To each her own.

This same woman wrote blithely about the length of her bowel movements which she measured each day to assess the state of her health. Twelve inches of poop was OK, but 18 inches were a red-letter day, to be celebrated with public announcements. Floating lumps are better than ones that sink. Sunk lumps are better than none at all. Spare me. There has to be a better way of figuring out how you feel each day without sticking your head in the toilet bowl to measure, count and weigh the contents.

You could try iridology, for example. I did. Six scant weeks before I found the lump in my breast that sent me scurrying down the rabbit hole of tests, more tests, diagnosis, and the three-tier level of conventional treatment, I went to a natural healing clinic. The word "college" in its name lent it an air of credibility. It had been highly recommended by a friend who went every week for a variety of ailments, many of which she hadn't known she had until she started going to this place.

I was invited to drink natural spring water in the tiny waiting room, a nice touch, before being ushered into the office of a severe-looking woman wearing pince-nez and a frown. Her white lab coat was another nudge toward credibility. She had analysed my saliva samples already; now she studied my eyes with intensity.

Her diagnosis was that I had a problem with one ovary, and my thyroid gland was in deep trouble. Surely she was mixing me up with Jem, our dog, whose thyroid gland suddenly ran amok, inflating him into a 55-pound balloon of canine lethargy and incipient insanity. His normal weight — if anything about that dog can be called normal — was 22 pounds. He was put on people pills for the rest of his life to stabilize his malfunctioning gland. The druggist carefully marked the prescription "Jem DOG Williams" so that we couldn't claim them on our drug insurance plan.

But I wasn't exhibiting any of the symptoms Jem did; I wasn't diving through closed screen doors or into already occupied bathtubs when a loon cried out in the lake; I wasn't edging desperately into the fireplace at the blast of a firecracker out in the street — even when there was a fire blazing in the grate. However, Pince-Nez showed me proof — which I was not allowed to take away with me — a chart of the irises of my disbelieving eyes; the specks she'd pencilled in certain sectors of this badly photocopied master chart indicated the areas of "weakness" in my health. And she'd sprinkled a whole rash of specks in the thyroid sector. What more proof did I need?

That Other Place

I suppose it was only coincidence that my friend had received exactly the same diagnosis. There must have been a lot of thyroid going around that spring.

Pince-Nez told me about her own life, her personal conversion on the road to Damascus when she discovered natural healing. She could have taught Jimmy Swaggart a thing or two about proselytizing.

"I was at death's door, and now look at me."

I looked at her. This woman, you obeyed. What I saw was about the skinniest person I have ever seen close up.

"I've never felt better. I just hadn't realized how I was poisoning my body with the unhealthy stuff I was putting into it," she continued, her voice shrill with commitment.

She then went on to name all my favourite foods. Her skeletal frame suggested that not only was she not eating unhealthily, she wasn't eating at all.

"Do you have a microwave?" she asked, her brow creased with fervour, or maybe hunger.

"Yes," I answered proudly, relieved that I was doing something right.

"Get rid of it immediately," she ordered.

Rats, and I had just managed to replace all my aluminum saucepans with glass ones.

"Microwaves kill all the vitamins in food. It kills everything nutritious. You don't want to eat dead food, do you?"

On a scale of one to ten? Well, yes, if the alternative was eating live food, such as in mooing steaks, clucking chickens and lobsters ferociously snapping at my fork. Even vegetables and fruit are technically dead once they have been dug or picked. Unless of course she was suggesting that we all graze in orchards and gardens like a herd of cows, nibbling grasses as they grew.

She instructed me to replace my microwave with a juicer, not one of those cheap models you could pick up at Sears but the very best designer brand, which the "college" just happened to sell. It also sold vitamins, oils, herbs, lotions — so convenient. Like the sheep that I was, I bought a selection of vitamins from

On and Off the Bandwagons

her, all the time asking myself "What is wrong with this picture?" Which was not quite so bad as my friend Andy, who bought $80 worth of fibre tabs from a door-to-door salesman. They tasted like insulation. They were even the same colour, a bright unnatural pink. They probably *were* insulation. She claims that she doesn't feel drafts so much now ...

In Pince-Nez's long detailed account of all my health "weaknesses," there wasn't a whisper of cancer. Amazing, that a tumour could spring into being and metastasize all within six weeks. Or else I had lying eyes.

I went back to the "college" one more time for a special healing massage during which the masseuse nearly tore my head off in an attempt to stem the arthritis already in situ. I never returned.

Another mecca of good health I have managed to miss is macrobiotic cooking. It has been around for years but is still highly suspect. At least I highly suspect it, and so does the *Dictionary of Common Fallacies* which debunks all sorts of fascinating beliefs such as that children can grow gold teeth, the degenerate descendants of aliens live in Tibet and that one swallow makes a summer. Right up there with the single swallow and the gold teeth is the macrobiotic diet:

> Where Aristotle had to deal with those who believed in armomancy (a method by which his contemporaries deduced from a person's shoulders whether he or she was a fit sacrifice for the gods), we have to deal with cranks who try to convince everybody that one's diet should be balanced between *yin* and *yang* foods. It turns out that it is almost impossible to apply this meaningless principle beyond a fixed diet of whole grain cereal, and it becomes increasingly difficult to convince oneself that whole grain cereal and nothing but the grain cereal is a balanced diet ... For a balanced diet, ignore the 'balanced diet' fiends ... George Ohsawa ... propagate[s] the doctrine embodied in his book *Zen Macrobiotics* ... he states that a diet of 100% whole grain cereal and 'sips of liquid' will cure cancer." (p. 167)

Ohsawa throws in mental diseases, heart trouble and haemophilia for good measure.

I remember reading about a spate of deaths in the late 1960s of adherents to this diet; people literally starved to death on it. It seemed that they were mostly flaxen-haired families living in the hinterland of Vermont. The "sips of liquid" could be the essential element: I suppose these must include that old favourite, liquidized lettuce.

They certainly couldn't be martinis, because another book I read, from Britain, said that a woman with metastatic breast cancer "slowly adopted a macrobiotic diet by reducing her intake of red meat, dairy food, and martinis." There must be degrees of macrobiotic, then: this fastidious lady is now more macrobiotic than another who is still quaffing jugs of gin. It's all relative, I guess.

I hesitate even to discuss diet, let alone offer advice, because I set such a bad example. I agree with La Rochefoucauld, who said, "To suffer one's health at the cost of too strict a diet is a tiresome illness indeed." I went on binges of trying to follow all the edicts, most of which start with "remove coffee, tea, tobacco, alcohol, fats, dairy products, meat, salt, sugar and strong spices from your diet." I don't know a whole lot of people who eat tobacco, except maybe baseball players before they discovered bubble gum, but hey, why quibble. The meaning was clear. Stop eating and drinking. Which would indeed be a cure for cancer because you would be dead.

I don't think that is quite the goal in mind, although, as recently as 1973 there was a firm medical belief in the efficacy of starvation. The theory was that by feeding the patient, you fed the cancer too, that eating enhanced tumour growth, a no-win theory.

It was believed that the patient's body and the cancer itself were competing for food. (Bradley and Nass, p. 148) However, there is overwhelming evidence that you won't encourage tumour growth by eating well. Exactly the opposite. One school of thought contends that tumours grow at a maximal rate regardless of nutrient intake, which means that it depletes your store of nutrients at a certain rate regardless of replenishment. "If you do not replace the nutrients the cancer cell has hoarded, you are likely to die of the side effects of starvation." (*Ibid.*, p. 149)

If you starve, you won't be around long enough to suffer the side effects. But the meaning is clear, despite the oddity of explanation: eat well to give yourself the strength to fight the cancer and to buy time to allow chemotherapy and radiation to do their thing.

In the medical mainstream, there still is not a whole lot of support for nutrition as more than back-up in cancer therapy. Some cancer clinics will refer you to a nutritionist if you ask, some won't. Mostly this area is given a cursory nod in the race to load the big guns of cancer treatment. Witness the hospital food that still is mostly inedible.

Eat well, yes; balance your meals with food from the four food groups; avoid too much fat, too much sugar. That was the extent of the nutritional advice I received from the clinic besides the one suggestion from my oncologist, which utterly endeared her to me.

"By all means, have a glass of wine if you feel like it, if you can keep it down. It won't kill you. It will relax you probably, which is just what you need."

Why I was worrying about a glass of wine with all the toxic waste swirling inside me from chemo, I'm not sure. A case of wonky perspective again.

Another piece of advice made eminent sense. My GP suggested that I record everything I ate for a week, every single thing I put in my mouth, to establish "base data." What it did was shock me right out of my smug assumption that I was eating healthily, except for too much coffee. I found this pathetic record in an old diary; it peters out after two entries, and no wonder.

October 29: 4 cups coffee
bowl of granola with milk
2 pieces of toast with bacon

That Other Place

2 glasses orange juice
roast beef sandwich (large) [written in tiny letters]
brownie
date square
macaroni cheese and hot dog in bun
small portion [written in large letters] cheesecake
2 glasses milk

October 30: 3 cups coffee
1 glass apple juice
2 pieces cracked wheat toast and peanut butter
apple
small cup of chicken soup
all-beef hot dog and bun
2 glasses wine

After two days I didn't want to play any more. It was too depressing; that was the end of the record. Already, on the second day I was getting defensive — *all-beef* hot dog, for godsake. And this from a person who would have claimed that she never ate hot dogs.

In the early weeks of surgery and chemo I lost 15 pounds — actually I think I shed them all in about two days — fear is very thinning. So I was never tempted to return to the cabbage diet which we all had tried with varying degrees of success the year before. It was a seven-day affair, a strange ruthless diet starting with only fruit, second day only vegetables, third day both, fourth day six bananas and six glasses of skim milk, fifth day tomatoes and beef, sixth and seventh day I forget because I never made it that far.

It was called the cabbage diet because the days were punctuated with steamy bowls of liquid swamp you made yourself carefully following the recipe that said: "cut up two cabbages, five onions, add water, salt and pepper, cook and eat as much as you want." Safe to say, because after the first bowlful you did not want. Well, not actually true because by the banana day you would eat anything.

On and Off the Bandwagons

We all tried this diet; it became a kind of refrain in our conversation. Andy left a message on my telephone answering machine one afternoon, identifying herself only as "cabbage breath." It was enough.

Sue and Seaton invited us for dinner one Friday night in the middle of yet another run at this diet.

"Oh, we can't come this week," I told Sue. "We are on the cabbage diet, and on Friday we can only eat tomatoes and beef."

"So are we," she said. "Come over and we'll share."

We shared all right. A seven-pound roast of beef and about a bushel of tomatoes among the four of us. My nephew, John, had designs on the leftovers and came in later that evening to a beef bone picked clean.

"I don't believe you guys ate the whole thing," he said in sorrowful astonishment. Neither could we. We lay about replete, and sozzled from the many glasses of wine that we deemed essential to survive the cabbage purge. It was about then it dawned on us that the five or six pounds we would lose in the week would be right back in about three days.

Some of the cancer diets are more understanding than others. I particularly liked the approach of one sent to me by a friend in Dublin. It was entitled "Cancer — Nutrition and Detoxification," compiled by Dr. B and the *late* Dr. A. This was not an auspicious start. It demoted coffee from a beverage to an enema, something that struck me as very Irish. Another of its edicts had a pronounced schizophrenic ring to it: "Alcohol, tea, coffee, chocolate and tobacco should be TOTALLY forbidden. Alcohol is forbidden for those with liver cancer as the liver has to de-toxicate it and would probably not be able to cope. However, alcohol (ethyl) at 30 mgm% begins to stimulate protaglandin formation. With the exception of those with liver cancer therefore, a hot toddy at night is permissible." I lived in Ireland for six years, and after the first year of reeling with culture shock I grew to love the country and its people with their endearing, frustrating, slightly skewed approach to almost everything. It was with glee that I encountered it again in the late Dr. A.'s humane and permissive prescription.

That Other Place

Quite a different emotion rocked me when I read a horrific little booklet I picked up in a drug store in Arizona, entitled "Avoiding Cancer Nature's Way." For the first time I began to feel an urge to support censorship. Right up there with fire and brimstone, this little screed was scaremongering of the worst kind. Packed into it was enough guilt-tripping to curdle the reader into total inertia and an early demise.

"Doctors say that over eighty percent of all cancers come from things we do to ourselves ... In most cases cancer is something we bring upon ourselves." Thank you.

It summed up conventional treatment in one contemptuous paragraph: "There's chemotherapy, which leaves you sick, weak and hairless. Surgery can cut the tumors out of your body, but that may not stop them from returning somewhere else. Massive doses of powerful drugs and radiation treatment are used to kill the cancer, but again there's no guarantee that the 'growing mechanism' has been shut down permanently."

The vision is of a tumour stealthily crawling down a hospital hallway from the surgery waste basket, slithering into your room, up onto the bed and nestling right back down into your breast, liver, brain, wherever.

It goes on to give holistic treatments a thoroughly bad name by espousing them. In a cloud of inaccuracy, wild claims and excruciating writing, the author intones: "Preventing cancer is as simple as changing your diet, say the experts." Would that it were so. And how is this for a heading: "Smoking and Emotions: Both Can Kill." Give up both and presumably you will live a long life. Notice the absence of "and happy" life, since emotions are taboo. But then a few pages later, "Can I Think Away Cancer? Medical research seems to say 'yes, you can.' All that is needed is a positive attitude, a joy for life, and a desire to live." Reading on, you discover that in fact you have not caused your own cancer because either your mother or your house did, one through thoughtlessly passing on the wrong genetic make-up, the other through radon, asbestos and formaldehyde. So you heave a sigh of relief, cast away the guilts, only to be nailed again with the huckster screech on the back cover: "Beating Cancer! The word strikes fear in us all. Yet we bring most kinds of cancer on ourselves. WE can win if we obey the rules of good living. Read them all inside."

This indeed is a freak show of a book.

I found and read this little piece of rubbish when I was feeling fairly strong, both mentally and physically. If I had seen it during the dark days of diagnosis and treatment, its facile message would have been really destructive. For instance, how would I have reacted to this description of breast cancer and its simplistic cause: "Imagine that a cancerous tumor is a plant growing inside your body. Imagine its roots growing inside your organs, wrapping around your liver and penetrating one of your kidneys. If that plant were left unwatered and unfed, it, like any other house plant, would soon die. So what keeps the deadly cancer plant well-fed and well-watered inside your body? Fat does."

Period. As simple as that? Give me a break.

Luckily there is the right kind of literature out there, exciting, door-opening books that counteract this sort of tripe. Informative, balanced studies in alternative treatments of cancer are inching their way into the medical mainstream.

-XX-
Is There a Cancer Personality?

There is smoke but no fire in those data.
Oncologist on CBC Radio, "Ideas," 1992

Stalking the pages of much of the literature on cancer therapy, both the good and the loony, is the cancer personality. It has been spawned by the "personalization" of disease that Susan Sontag objects to so strenuously. She perceives the cancer personality as simply an updated version of the tuberculosis personality, asserting that it was with TB that the idea of individual illness was articulated, that a disease was perceived to match a personality. Wherever it came from it causes much discussion.

There are Type A personalities and Type B personalities; these seem to have gained acceptance as real. Type As are the aggressive, strong-willed, choleric workaholics who are prone to heart attacks. The Bs are quieter, less competitive, laid back and not prone to heart attacks. And now there is the Type C personality — people who are passive, who suppress anger, who cope, who pride themselves on coping and for their pains often end up with cancer.

I don't think C stands for Cancer, or for Coping, but it might. It also could stand for Credulous, Cadaver or Calamity. This theory has found its way into the popular press, which means that it is somewhat simplified, somewhat distorted and, as a result, somewhat suspect.

Is There a Cancer Personality?

The cancer personality theory began to crop up as early as the 1950s; one physician declared that the patients with the fastest growing tumours had "serious, overcooperative, overnice, overanxious, painfully sensitive, passive, apologetic personalities." (Barber, p. 96) This is the kind of observation designed to give cancer patients a bad name and a horrendous guilt complex. It also is probably the foundation for the skewed logic expressed by a hospital administrator in Vancouver, 25 years later. A delegation had gone to complain about the scheduling procedures followed by the cancer clinic which may have been easier to organize but resulted in long waits for patients.

The administrator's response? "But cancer patients like to wait," he said, and with a figurative pat on the head sent the delegation packing.

But then, what about our reputation as shit-disturbers: "Cancer patients are notoriously difficult to please, doctors and nurses have told me. We are, these caregivers say, an angry group. We demand care and attention. We are often uncooperative. We complain." (Johnson, p. 86) So now we are schizophrenics, already?

Maybe we are just people first, individuals with loves, hates, personality traits just like everyone else who isn't struggling in the maw of illness and its concomitant treatment. We are cancer patients second, with all the trappings of various interpretations of the C personality; and then there is that third unfortunate category —The Disease — favoured by the Blitskis of the world, scientists whose reality is only what they see under a microscope.

It is hard for doctors, administrators and nurses to remember; it is often hard for us cancer patients ourselves to remember. You begin to see yourself through a glass darkly, the wavy distortions of illness clouding the person that used to be you before you became an illness.

All these personality theories — cancer, TB, heart, etc. — actually support the erosion of individuality with their general sweep of all those suffering from a particular disease into one pigeonhole.

That Other Place

When tuberculosis was on the rampage, before it was nearly eradicated by the discovery of antibiotics, there was a tuberculosis personality. TB sufferers, in literature at least, are depicted as sensitive, passive people who lack the will to survive. They may be passionate, artistic types but they all appear to suffer from a major lack of vitality. This romantic notion overlooks one little thing. It was not just the Camilles who succumbed to tuberculosis. Consumption felled artists and writers, yes. It also felled people from every other walk of life, especially those who didn't get enough to eat, whose houses, if they had houses, were damp and cold. It attacked whole populations of Inuit when they were exposed to "white man's" diseases, not because they were passive artists, but because their bodies had no immunities built up against the disease.

Talk of a consumptive personality disappeared with the almost total eradication of the disease, and has not reappeared with the recent advent of a frightening strain of tuberculosis that is resisting antibiotics. With the disease-personality theory, it is the old cause-and-effect conundrum: which comes first, the illness or the personality that comes to be associated with it, the cancer or the chicken that gets it? Does cancer kick into existence a particular passive, coping response? Or is a passive, suppressed personality the lightning rod that attracts the disease like a heat-detecting missile zooming in on a cauldron of repressed emotion?

It seems more likely that a cancer diagnosis begins the spiral of fear and depression and suppression which helps to break down the immune system even further. The *reputation* of the disease is part of its deadly nature. If we responded to a diagnosis of cancer the same way we react to a diagnosis of flu, perhaps there would be more survivors? Sontag touches on this when she complains of the negative power of cancer as metaphor.

The cancer personality theory, which has been contested and debated for 30 years, appears to be a corollary of the assumption that stress is one of the main culprits in the genesis of a cancer. People who are passive and stoic, who put other

Is There a Cancer Personality?

people's needs before their own, are repressing their emotions; this repressive trait disarms them in the battle to handle stress. They bottle up everything inside and eventually implode. The emotions caused by stress are internalized and weaken the immune system to such an extent that it can no longer protect the person from physical illness.

Studies have shown that people who are under emotional stress have a much higher rate of ailments, ranging from common colds to terminal illness. These are not just psychosomatic illnesses, but ones that so far have not been linked with anything other than a bacteria or virus — a physical cause. The theory goes that those people who express their emotions — Type A personalities — get rid of stress or handle it by externalizing their emotions, thus protecting or strengthening their immune systems and fending off illness.

The studies are somewhat fuzzy because so many of them rely on patients' assessments of themselves, by necessity, *after* they have been diagnosed with an illness. The perspective provided from inside a disease is not always the clearest.

When I first heard about the cancer personality, I was astounded at how it matched mine — passive, compliant, coping, anxious to please. I tried out my theory on Allen.

"You, passive? " He rolled his eyes in disbelief. "What? Are you on drugs?"

I was stung. Did he forget, I was doing several lines of chemotherapy at the time?

"Tell me when you have been passive and compliant. Tell me when, just one instance."

"Yah, well there were lots of times." My theory wasn't holding up very well. "And I *am* good at coping."

"What has coping got to do with suppressing emotion, with being compliant? Doesn't it just mean that you might be innovative at dealing with whatever comes up? You coped with the flood in the office last summer. The power was off, the sump pump didn't work, the rains came down, the basement filled up with water and you coped. You went out into the storm, you drove along sidewalks to avoid the rivers flowing down Island

That Other Place

Park Drive and you borrowed a gas generator from a store that does not lend, only sells, gas generators. And then you got me to come home and bail. That's coping. Does that mean you are more susceptible to cancer than a person who would have just sat in the rising water, drumming their heels and throwing a tantrum?"

"I think my theory needs some work."

Further reading, months later, clarified the "coping aspect" of the cancer personality. It seems there is "coping" and then there is "coping." One is a good way of resolving difficulties, of adjusting successfully to external influences apparently beyond your control. This fits exactly with the dictionary definition — "to struggle or contend, esp. on fairly even terms or with some degree of success." The not-so-good way of coping is the one bound up in the definitions of a cancer personality —it's coping by resignation, by making do.

Not only was I not such a great example of the cancer personality, I have yet to encounter one among all the people I have met in the last five years who had or has cancer. Maybe I've been hanging out with the wrong type of cancer patient. For instance, how does Stella fit? Here is a woman who got breast cancer, and if that wasn't enough, then had a heart attack. So now she not only has to cope with two major diseases, she has to deal with a split personality?

Stella does say that the atmosphere in the waiting room at the Heart Institute is quite different from that of the cancer clinic. Choleric, overweight, impatient men apparently pace up and down seething at having to wait more than five minutes to see their doctors. They send their wives down to put more money in the parking meters, wives who are usually small, quiet and passive. Potential cancer sites, obviously.

Stella pointed out that in the cancer waiting room, hardly anyone seethes or paces, and it is the patient, not the spouse, who struggles out to put money in the meter.

And here is a thought: at the Civic Hospital in Ottawa, the cancer clinic has about 12 assigned parking spots. The Heart Institute has a whole block-long parking lot. The Heart Institute

Is There a Cancer Personality?

has its own building; the cancer clinic is tucked into the back of the hospital. April is cancer month; the Heart Foundation holds its fund-raising telethon the first week in April. Seems to be some evidence here underlying the personality theory after all. Those tough, aggressive, heart patients do not accept second best; they raise money, enlist volunteers, take over parking areas with a will. Apparently cancer patients do not attack with the same panache; perhaps they are too busy surviving.

Support for the cancer personality theory waxed and waned throughout the 1970s and 1980s but it appears to be enjoying a revival. In 1987, at the University of California, a psychologist, Lydia Temoshok, recast the cancer personality as a particular "coping style" that she felt characterized many of the 150 melanoma patients she studied at a local clinic. "Compared with the classic Type A personality — hard-driving, choleric and susceptible to heart attacks — many of the melanoma patients were passive, compliant and reluctant or unable to express emotion ... [A]fter classifying and placing each patient ... she found that immune activity was highest in the bodies of the patients who expressed more emotion." (Barber, p. 99)

Even *The Canadian Breast Cancer Series*, published in 1988 by the YM-YWCA of Winnipeg, a very straight, informative, no-nonsense study, gives the personality theory a nod:

> The role of personality traits in the development of breast cancer is an area of conflicting reports. Hypothetically, suppression of emotion may lead to a biological response which increases risk of cancer. This would seem to indicate a need to monitor your breasts if you are the type of person who is patient, unassertive or unable to express anger. (p. 64)

How about expressing laughter? That quote prickles with the embattled words of authors cornered by a committee which has wrenched the sense right out of the paragraphs in its attempt to sit on the fence. It is trying to toe the straight medical line while giving the nod to what it considers slightly off-the-wall theories. I have written for committees and I recognize the tell-tale traces of many, many drafts in this beleaguered prose. Some committee members said, leave out the personality schtick, it's all hokum; others said, put it in, cancer is a disease of the personality. The authors' heads swing like yoyos, and the result is that image of a poor repressed recluse crouched in a corner, "monitoring" her breasts with fixed intensity, waiting for the suppressed emotions to pop up on them like mushrooms.

This theory should carry a warning with it, though: innocent bystanders beware; repressed passions — other people's — could be damaging to your health. After stabbing his wife, Norman Mailer apparently justified his action by claiming that if he hadn't allowed expression of his "murderous nest of feeling" he would have developed cancer and died within a few years himself. Yikes.

One of the troubles with the personality theory, aside from its questionable ancestors, is the guilt it can create. It's bad enough to have cancer, without having to feel guilty about it. The three-o'clock-in-the-morning thoughts, what my father called "The Horrifications," are the ones that plunge you into guilt and despair. "If I had only lashed out when I was angry, if I hadn't been such a door mat, if I just hadn't coped! If! If! If! Then I wouldn't have cancer today."

This way lies madness, which is the direction of all thoughts roaming the Horrification hours just before dawn.

And it doesn't matter when the proponents of such theories say, "Of course you shouldn't blame yourself, it's not your fault. Don't take it personally. It's just your personality." As Renate Rubinstein demands so indignantly, "Well, I ask you, what can be more personal than your personality?"

-XXI-
Taking Control

*Meditation may be the therapeutic tool
capable of unsticking the body from the disease.*

Deepak Chopra, *Quantum Healing*

Centuries ago, in most cultures including our own, the connection between emotions and physical health was recognized and accepted. Somewhere along the line, Western medicine abandoned this connection in favour of purely chemical and physical cause and effect. But we are coming full circle with a growing school of thought confirming that connection again. For the sceptics, there is even scientific proof: the relationship between mind and body can now be confirmed by tracing nervous and chemical reactions within the body in response to emotional states. The bridge between emotions and health seems to be the immune system.

In the last 15 years, knowledge of how the nerves work has changed dramatically; it used to be thought that they transmitted messages through electric impulses; however, in the 1970s, the discovery of neuro-transmitters, a new class of minute chemicals, has begun to lift the curtain on the mystery of the relationship between mind and body. It seems that the impulse sent by the mind to the body is chemical, not electrical, in nature.

The discovery of brain chemicals, called monocytes, in the immune system suggests that intelligence floats freely through the body — that the brain does not relate to the body only on fixed systems such as the nervous system. The immune system apparently sends and receives messages that are just as diverse as the messages transmitted by neurons.

Psychoneuroimmunology is the name of this fast-growing field of study of the connection between emotions and physical well-being.

> At the very instant that you think, 'I am happy,' a chemical messenger translates your emotion, which has no solid existence whatever in the material world, into a bit of matter so perfectly attuned to your desire that literally every cell in your body learns of your happiness and joins in. The fact that you can instantly talk to 50 trillion cells in their own language is just as inexplicable as the moment when nature created the first photon out of empty space. (Chopra, p. 127)

Norman Cousins was one of the first to bring to the attention of the general public the theory that the right kind of emotion can actually make you better — not just *feel* better. In his groundbreaking book, *Anatomy of an Illness*, he describes how he checked himself out of hospital and into a hotel, and watched old Marx brothers movies and segments of "Candid Camera." His laughter eased his pain to the point where he could cut way back on painkillers, and ultimately, he believes, helped boost his immune system to such an extent that he recovered from an incurable illness. He has since done it a second time.

Even though out of his whole book, only about one and a half pages were devoted to laughter, now, 15 years later, Cousins is still known as the person who cured himself of a terminal illness by laughing himself well. He has tried to clear up this misconception many times. In 1985 he and another doctor even took out a full-page ad in the *Los Angeles Times* to try and correct the misinterpretation of his statements. But the sad fact is, he is probably responsible, albeit inadvertently, for the revolting description of laughter as "internal jogging," a term that casts it into the stewpot of self-improvement techniques. It's right up there with "dork walking," yoghurt and bean sprouts. In some circles laughter has become a duty; next step religion.

Taking Control

It's fascinating that that one small reference to the curative powers of laughter has been pounced on by so many people. The idea is obviously very appealing, but this abbreviated interpretation leaves out the most important link, just as the statement "stress causes cancer" does.

> Laughter in and of itself cannot cure cancer nor prevent cancer, but laughter as part of the full range of positive emotions including hope, love, faith, strong will to live, determination and purpose, can be a significant and indispensable aspect of the total fight for recovery. (Cousins, p. 130)

୪୦

About two months into chemotherapy, I sat in my usual spot in the ante-room of the blood-test room at the clinic, idly listening in on a conversation between the two women beside me. One, the picture of health with glowing skin and smile, was telling the other about a self-help group for cancer patients in Ottawa.

Had I heard this conversation even as much as two weeks before, I would have paid scant attention. Until then I wanted only the printed word as my travelling companion, and I wanted only "facts" — statistics that I was on the right side of, terse descriptions of new treatment from the Cancerline data base, medical explanations of the disease, individual accounts of experience with chemotherapy, surgical procedures similar to mine, a shopping bag full of pamphlets and booklets from the cancer clinic. Any other writing on the subject I viewed with suspicion; no one was going to trick me into being positive about this whole wretched business.

My angry rejection of the video of beautiful, articulate women telling how they had "beaten" cancer had not been because of its content but because of timing; I couldn't see it except through a haze of disbelief and pessimism, which turned the smiling earnest faces of cancer survivors into egregious tricksters.

I didn't want to talk to any other patient; I didn't want to "share"; I wanted to stump along alone; well, alone except for my own personal support group of Allen, Matt, Sam, my brothers and sisters-in-law, my father, my step-children, close friends, all who wove a skein of love and help about me. But alone in the sense that I was the only traveller; my family and friends cheered and encouraged from the border. And without them I wouldn't have cleared the first hurdle.

For some reason that day I broke out of my self-imposed constrictions and approached one of the women in the clinic foyer. My conversation with her set me off on a new path through this desert country, one that teemed with fellow travellers, and in a direction that has helped immeasurably since those first rudderless months following diagnosis.

It led to the discovery of a whole new layer of treatment — one that gave me some control because it was initiated and developed by me. I learned how to enlist my mind and emotions in the fight against cancer; in a figurative sense I was the one wielding the scalpel, the needle, the radiation ray through the non-invasive, benign interference of my own brain. What a revelation, what a gift.

This conversation also introduced me to a small coterie of cancer patients in Ottawa who had formed a self-help therapy group — Mind Over Cancer. It was such a release, to talk to other people who had cancer, to share experiences, to laugh together — oh the humour, so black, so funny and so unshareable except with people in the same predicament; to let down barriers, to allow the bright silly smile you wore for most of the world to slide away, and find it replaced with a real smile, because there was no need for pretence. There was such pain too, because no matter how hard people try, some still do die of cancer.

The woman with the look of glowing health, Jeannie, scribbled a note on a piece of paper just before she went down the hall to see her oncologist. It turned out that she was not the "support person," as I had assumed, but a cancer patient herself. The note said, "Have you read Simonton or Bernie Siegel?"

Simonton I knew about: I had three copies of *Getting Well*

Again and his cassette tape, all given to me by friends; they lay gathering dust on my bedside table. I thought Siegel was a baseball player. Did he write books too?

This bit of paper was a passport into a new world, the two names a cypher with which to break the code that had blocked my earlier, feeble attempts to understand. Suddenly there was a wealth of writing and an approach to cancer I had earlier rejected through a miasma of fear, cynicism and inertia.

I had started Simonton's book in the very early days but had abandoned it after a few pages. It opens with "Everyone participates in his or her health or illness at all times. This book will show people with cancer or other serious illnesses how they can participate in getting well again." Right away, it had two strikes against it: it appeared to be saying that it was my fault that I had cancer, and to get better I would have to work at it. The whole idea of doing anything other than follow doctors' orders fatigued and irritated me. And I had enough guilt without the added zinger of being held responsible for getting sick and maybe dying sooner than I should.

It had been the wrong time for me to read this book: the shock and fright of cancer, the pain of surgery and the growing nausea of chemo all stood between me and the opening words that had probably been carefully chosen, but not carefully enough. I found them offensive. After Jeannie's note, I gave the book another try. When *Getting Well Again* was first published in 1978, its premise was a revelation — the idea that a person's reaction to stress and other emotional factors can contribute to the onset and progress of cancer; that the will to live can translate into a physical response to disease. It is still considered revolutionary, by many.

Carl Simonton and his then wife Stephanie Matthews-Simonton had been working in this area since 1969. As a cancer specialist at the University of Oregon Medical School, Simonton started tracking the correlation between longer survival and a specific goal. Some patients, who claimed that indeed they wanted to live, continued to undermine their stated desire with actions that ensured that they couldn't get well. For example, people with lung cancer continued to smoke; people with liver cancer continued to drink heavily. But some patients who had been sent home after minimal treatment, with a life-expectancy of zero, were surviving for years, apparently healthy and symptom-free. The Simontons wanted to know why.

The common thread in the data gathered on those survivors who were inexplicably beating the statistics was their expression of a goal. They all wanted to live, not forever but long enough to write a book, to see a son or daughter graduate, to see and hear, one more time, the geese flying south for the winter, even something as simple as moving and settling in another town. So they did.

Bernie Siegel tells of one of his patients who was determined to survive her particularly virulent cancer until her daughter got married. A few years later her daughter took a husband, but the mother did not die. At a subsequent check-up, Siegel asked her why not? She said craftily, "Hey, you forget, I have another daughter."

In 1990, Dr. David Phillips from the University of California, San Diego, did a statistical study of death certificates of people from two cultures, Jewish and Chinese, before and after an important festivity in each religion — Passover and the Harvest Moon Festival. He discovered that the death rate fell 24 percent among the Jewish community just before Passover, and rose 24 percent immediately afterward. In the Chinese community the death rate fell by 35 percent before the Harvest Moon Festival and rose 35 percent directly afterward. It appeared that a lot of people were hanging in there to enjoy the festivities before shuffling off this mortal coil.

The death certificates studied were those of people who died through natural causes, not "external" ones as Phillips put it, an odd term describing death by suicide, homicide or accident. The rates of slow-down were highest for stroke victims, then heart attacks, then cancer, ostensibly a disease whose outcome could not be influenced by psychological means.

Dr. Phillips is careful not to make any claims regarding the connection between mind and body, nor does he comment on the astonishing match of percentages before and after the anticipated event. What he did was throw the ball squarely into the medical court: this is what the statisticians have found; now it is up to you, you doctors, to confirm, explain or refute the findings with your own medical control studies.

In the meantime, this study is one more nail in the coffin of belief that cancer — or any other disease — is strictly physical. It suggests that the will to live is not just a mechanism used by a novelist to propel the plot along, not just an apocryphal element of family lore that tells of an aged great aunt belligerently hanging on for years with the sole purpose of preventing her son from throwing himself away on that young guttersnipe from the wrong side of town. Not necessarily a conscious act, it seems to be something in the mind that kicks in when an individual's life is threatened, an entity which must lurk right along there with the soul, the intelligence and the cells' memories.

Much of the literature on alternative medicine acknowledges the seminal research of the Simontons. They were the first Western medical doctors to involve the patient's help in his or her own cancer treatment through the mobilization of the mind. With startling success, they taught patients how to use visualization, meditation and relaxation, the three big guns of mind/body medicine, as techniques to strengthen their immune systems against illness.

Surgery, chemo and radiation concentrate solely on the physical ramifications of the disease; visualization, meditation and relaxation techniques enlist the mind, both the conscious and the subconscious, in eradicating cancer from the body. At the same time these techniques are directed at eliminating the possible causes, as well as the symptoms, of the disease.

In *Quantum Healing*, Chopra writes in frustration:

> [T]he underlying philosophy in cancer treatment is that the mind will just have to stand by while the body endures devastation. In other words, an open clash is actually encouraged in the mind-body system. How can this be called healing? In a clash between mind and body, the patient is fighting on both sides — there is

only his body and his mind. Isn't it obvious that when a loser emerges, it will be he? (p. 265)

Made sense to me. If there was a way of persuading my mind to work *with* the physical treatments that appeared to wreak havoc, then I was all for it. At first though, it was hard to make connections. So I relax, so I meditate, so what? How can these activities have a physical response? Yes, I want to live, but how does this desire, no matter how powerful, translate into a cure or even a delay in the progression of the disease?

These are the tools that allow you to reach emotions, to direct the forces of the mind — an enormous arsenal — on the body.

Relaxation, the necessary first step to reach the other two techniques, allows you to let go of the tension, both physical and mental; it creates the environment for connections. Relaxation techniques vary from person to person and become easier with practice. These aren't the relaxations of leisure — reading a good book, swimming, walking, going to a movie — although all those are just fine too, but the concentrated activities of letting go — consciously relaxing each muscle, each organ, including the brain.

Visualization is a way of mobilizing the imagination in combatting disease. By conjuring up actual scenes, you bring the mind in as an ally, directing the power of the imagination in a specific way.

Meditation is a state of mind achieved through relaxation; it is a sort of cleansing of the consciousness to reach the unconsciousness. Chopra calls it "diving through the gaps of your thoughts" to another plane altogether. Studies have proven that it can have profound effects on the physical body; through meditation, Eastern yogis can block pain, deny hunger, go without sleep beyond present Western understanding. In 1967, the first recent Western research proved these observations through controlled studies indicating that meditation can slow the heartbeat and decrease oxygen consumption. The subjects of the study had entered a state of deep and total relaxation but were completely alert. They had entered what some scientists call the fourth dimension (not waking, not sleeping and not dreaming). However, the body/mind approach to cancer treatment, through relaxation, meditation and visualization, is still on the suspect list in Canada. Despite growing evidence of its power and effectiveness, the doors of conventional medicine remain largely shut.

July 1990
Sylvia is dying. She is in the palliative care unit at the Queensway Carleton and the cancer has spread into her intestines, closed down the whole digestive system. She hasn't really eaten anything for weeks, only a little watermelon juice which she must not swallow. She grows thinner and more beautiful each day. Her voice is reedy now; she made a passing reference to the fact that she didn't have a voice anymore. Her courage and grace are overwhelming.

She asked today would my book include what no others have. What is that, I asked, full of sadness and admiration of her dignity and grace so close to the end of her life.

"No books tell you how to leave," she said. "Will yours?"

I desperately wanted to say yes, I wanted to tell her what she needed to know. But no, my book wouldn't have that, because I don't know how to leave either. No one does.

In the face of Sylvia's reality, all the theories and research, all the pat words of comfort and advice, the Kübler-Ross stages, the biblical texts, the jokes, the self-help proselytising, all wizen and die. All I could offer was my love and deep respect for Sylvia's way of leaving.

-XXII-
Mind/Body Medicine: Dealing with the Guilt

More people have died from religion than cancer.

Anon.

So many theories about cancer and its treatments throng this overly charted country, who is to say that one is more valid than another. New "findings" pop up every day, new versions, new approaches, and so often contradictory. It is a thoroughly confusing world both for patients and medical practitioners. For example, recent studies have established that oncogenes are present in everyone. They act like switches in the body's mechanism: if switched off they behave like normal cells. If switched on, they begin to grow and multiply in an abnormal fashion — they become cancer cells. The big question is what switches them on, and how can we learn to keep them turned off?

In the summer of 1990, a team of scientists in Australia announced a breakthrough in this area: they claimed to have reversed the growth of cancer cells by "switching off" the gene that caused the disease. A genetic engineering process developed by this group worked so dramatically and so thoroughly that all the cancer cells in the lab culture dish were quickly restored to a benign state. My usual response to the almost weekly announcements of new cancer cures is somewhat jaded now, but this one I read with excitement. The author of the article must have been a war correspondent looking for a war to report: "The five-person team introduced a gene close to a cancer-causing oncogene and used a biochemical trigger to stimulate it. This provoked a battle between the two in which the quiescent gene deformed the rogue oncogene and rendered it inactive." Sounds like a report from the Pentagon.

However, other "experts" from within the mainstream medical community raced forward with neon signs flashing "caution," or maybe "professional jealousy," and said huffily, that this was not the first time scientists have been able to turn off cancer genes, or at least to make them *look* normal. The ability to introduce foreign genes into every cancerous cell in the body is "a long way off, maybe never," according to one doctor at the Princess Margaret Hospital in Toronto who went on to stomp on already dashed hopes by adding, "It's a big leap" from the lab dish to humans. (*Ottawa Citizen*, Scientists claim breakthrough ...", 1990)

Of course it's a big leap, but isn't that what medical research is all about — the big leap? However, his caution is well-founded I guess, given the myriad cancer cures that bloom and die along the highways of this country. Out there in the middle of the road, we are easy targets for all the juggernauts with their cargo of conflicting cancer theories to plough us down.

The Western medical pundits really close ranks though on alternative medicine theories and treatments. Anything other than the purely physical and the thoroughly "proven" methods they tend to cast into the pale of crazy, dangerous or useless theories. Practitioners argue that non-traditional methods only offer false hope, and often financially bankrupt the patient because of their high costs.

Some do, there is no question. Made vulnerable and desperate by fear and pain, people with life-threatening illnesses will often chase down any path no matter how weird, dangerous, difficult or expensive. They will choose these routes sometimes as well as conventional treatment, sometimes instead of. Often they travel more alone than ever because of the incredulity of family and friends, which leaves them even more vulnerable to the loonies offering succour along the way. But, and it is a big but, to label everything but the standard cancer treatments of surgery, drugs and radiation as quackery is to be blind to exciting and effective results in other areas.

Every oncologist, surgeon, radiologist, GP and psychologist I have talked to about cancer emphasizes its unpredictability. Only Doc, the radiologist who helped with my decision whether to have radiation therapy, took the logical next step to admit, with a tinge of despair, "There are no experts in cancer. If anyone tells you he is an expert, do not believe him. There is no such thing." Which might explain why there are not a lot of phone-in shows on how to deal with cancer. There are expert gardeners telling you how to keep your roses aphid-free; there are expert vets who explain why your dog tries to bury bones in the living-room rug; there are even expert dentists who tell you that there really is no difference between caps and crowns — that you'll need to mortgage the farm to get either.

But there are no shows which you can phone and say, "Hello, Dr. X. I so enjoy your program, I listen to it every week. I have this cancer, and I simply can't get rid of it. I've tried everything, spraying it with defoliant, repotting it, even cutting it right back to nothing. It just keeps right on growing. What do you suggest? ... Dr. X? Dr. X.? Are you there?"

If he is, he is a charlatan. Tune him out at once — or her — because although they might not have Ask the Expert shows, there are doctors out there who claim to be experts and sell you nothing but a bill of goods, false hope and in some cases, a hastened death.

Surely the lack of experts, the unpredictability of the disease, the fact that after centuries of suffering, there is still no cure for breast cancer, no "magic bullets" like the Salk vaccine or insulin or penicillin, surely this sad state of medical affairs should encourage the medical community to explore more urgently beyond the confines of its physical treatments.

Time and again, certain directions in treatment beyond the conventional are proved efficacious. But Western medicine seems to blinker out the good with the bad, the exciting with the nutty, the possible with the dangerous. Take acupuncture, for example. When first introduced to North America it was met with howls of derision and scepticism from the Western medical world. Slowly, slowly, it is winning converts, at least with its results as a pain reliever and its success in treating addiction, although it's efficacy as an anaesthetic has been proven fallacious. Now, however, there are acupuncture clinics in most major cities in Canada; doctors from Western medical facilities are taking acupuncture courses, and the credentials of those doctors trained in acupuncture in China are being recognized here. Despite such acceptance, it is a treatment still not covered by Ontario's medical insurance plan, OHIP.

In 1989 in Quebec, a biologist, Gaston Naessens, was charged with illegal practice of medicine and contributing to the death of a woman, who, with metastasized breast cancer in the final stages, had refused all conventional treatment and had insisted on taking medicine developed by Naessens. Called 714-X, it was designed not to destroy cancer cells but to bolster the immune system and help the body heal itself. The patient had received injections of this substance, administered by a friend, for seven months before she died. The prosecution's case was that the woman might have survived if she had taken conventional treatment, and that Naessens knew his treatment to be worthless but that he hoped to profit from the desperation of someone in the throes of terminal illness.

The trial opened with a parade of doctors and scientists testifying to the "scientific untenability of 714-X and the spurious nature of Naessens' theories of cancer and its treatment." (Roberts, p. 52) Then witness after witness described the apparent cures they had achieved using Naessens' treatment. The testimonials to Naessens' integrity were overwhelming: "he'd never promised a cure, never told one of them to discontinue conventional treatment, and never asked for payment." (*Ibid.*, p. 54) Some sources described the trial as a "witch hunt." The jury delivered its verdict quickly: acquittal on all counts. Dr. Augustin Roy, head of the Quebec Medical Corporation, the professional self-regulating licensing body that had pushed for the charges to be laid, was quoted as saying that the trial was "wholly incomplete" and that the "patients who testified simply don't know the difference between *feeling* healthy and *being* healthy ... All of them should stand at attention or, more properly, get down on their knees to thank orthodox medicine for having kept them alive." (*Ibid.*) Apparently Roy didn't notice that most of Naessens' patients were refugees from conventional treatment. He did not give up there. Within weeks of the acquittal, 82 more counts of practising medicine without a licence were brought against Naessens, each carrying the possibility of a $5,000 fine. "As was clear from his rhetoric, Augustin Roy wasn't fighting any more to protect innocent patients from an unscrupulous quack. He was fighting to protect his profession from an alternative vision of healing." (*Ibid.*)

Unfortunately, there are dishonest or misguided people who make great claims for utterly useless or dangerous "cures" and these few give the whole area of alternative medicine a bad name. However, such "doctors" are not unknown to the corridors of traditional medicine either, something that conventional doctors seem to overlook in their haste to reject non-traditional methods of treatment. And as for costs, yes, some forms of alternative treatment are indeed costly for the patient because standard medical insurance will not cover them.

One of the criticisms of the theory that emotions, or the mind, can influence a physical disease is its sometime aura of guilt. If you can think yourself well, then the corollary is that you thought yourself sick. Stupid old you. Such a glib summary distorts the whole meaning of mind-body medicine, reducing it to an absurdity. Unfortunately much of the writing to come out of this area lends itself to such interpretation.

The Ontario Cancer Institute at the Princess Margaret Hospital in Toronto is the only research organization in Canada associated with a medical hospital, that specializes in mind/body healing techniques. In the spring of 1990, I spoke to the director of the Institute, Alastair Cunningham, and his executive assistant, Gwen Jenkins. I felt I already knew Dr. Cunningham from his imagery tapes — I had done the first segment of his course by then and

That Other Place

was eager to meet him for a number of reasons, not least that he is in the unique position of having been working in the field, working with cancer patients, exploring the mind/body connection long before he himself got cancer. He now has a foot in both camps.

I asked him if his approach had changed. Had his faith in self-help techniques withstood the crucible of his own cancer? He said that if anything, his personal disease strengthened his belief in the route he had already embarked on. "The general idea behind [this approach] is quite straightforward: if you have cancer, or indeed any chronic health problem, you can do a great deal to help yourself. Medical treatment remains the first line of defence in almost all cases, but you can augment its effects, and strengthen your body's natural defense mechanisms, with a variety of mental techniques and approaches." (Cunningham, introduction)

I asked him how he deals with the accusation that the coping techniques he teaches spawn self-blame in the cancer patient. He seemed bemused by the question, so far was he from the easy misunderstanding of the mind-over-illness approach.

"But that is irrelevant," he smiled, speaking slowly. "You feel guilty if you want. It has nothing to do with marshalling your mind, through meditation, relaxing, imagery, to fight the disease."

I wrestled with the guilt thing for months, particularly after a conversation with one woman who went at me and my pat proselytizing of mind/body stuff like a terrier at a bone.

I was visiting a friend in hospital. She had cancer — of course — and Donna arrived while I was there. Her husband was on another ward in the same hospital, with lymphoma. Did the whole world have cancer?

My friend set me up. "Pen's really interested in mind over cancer stuff and she's just back from a Bernie Siegel workshop," she said. "Ask her what she thought of him."

Donna said nothing, she just looked at me, waiting. Oblivious, I waded in. "It was a totally amazing experience — he's a charismatic presence, full of humour."

"I don't like him," Donna said flatly. "I don't believe his

Mind/Body Medicine: Dealing with the Guilt

message. It's harmful. I read his book and all it does is add guilt to misery."

I had read Siegel's books. By then I had been to two of his workshops, had read the Simontons' book and countless others on this very subject; I had listened to tapes, I was secretary of the Mind Over Cancer group in Ottawa, I had done Dr. Cunningham's courses; I had just returned from a week-long workshop on Cortes Island based on the mind/body connection in healing — and I couldn't answer her challenge.

"It's not anything to do with guilt, it's just fighting cancer with everything, not just physical treatment," I started lamely, listening to my own voice limp along, wondering what the hell I was going to say next.

"I found him a very funny man," was what I heard myself say. Wha ...? Donna's eyes dropped from my face, the eagerness fading. She wanted me to convince her. I had done nothing more than babble.

Two days later, something I read in Chopra's book, *Quantum Healing*, brought it all into focus for me. He described experiments in which incubated cold viruses were placed directly in the mucous lining of the nose: the owners of the noses came down with a cold only *12 percent of the time*. "These odds could not be increased by exposing the subjects to cold drafts, putting their feet into ice water to give them chills, or anything else that was purely physical." (p. 142) Why didn't they all get colds? According to the rules of physical medicine they should have. The reason had to lie in something other than the physical state of the noses and their owners.

Control studies have proven that, for example, loneliness improves a person's chances of developing cancer. It is recognized as a risk factor, just as smoking is a risk factor for lung cancer. But, just as is the case of physical carcinogens, not everyone who is lonely dies of cancer. Nor does every worker in an asbestos factory succumb to cancer. Each person is the sum of his or her experience. You are what you eat, was the trendy battle cry of the 1980s nutritionists. You are also what you feel, think, see, hear, do, don't do.

"The minutes of life silently accumulate, and like grains of sand deposited by a river, the minutes can eventually pile up into a hidden formation that crops above the surface as a disease." (*Ibid.*) The operable word in that quote is "can." Well, to be grammatically pure, it should be "may," suggesting cosmic as well as physical possibility. It is what each of us do with our experience that is unquantifiable, unmeasurable, unpredictable except in the broadest sense.

I developed breast cancer. Why? Not the raging, clenched-fist "Why me, God?" demand, but the rhetorical query that neither medical science, quantum physics nor human knowledge in any realm can answer yet. Why did only some of those noses develop colds? Aside from their physical state, there are elements we are not taking into consideration. Perhaps propensity for disease is influenced by the intelligence in the body cells that Chopra talks of, perhaps it is random fate, perhaps it is the individual's immune system, subconscious, emotions or genes. We don't really know.

What is increasingly evident is that the human mind has an enormous influence over "physical disease." To try and influence your physical state through your mind — on the simplest level through meditation, visualization imagery, even good old positive thinking as long as it is honest positive thinking, and not pure denial — does not presuppose the twisted corollary that you must have thought yourself sick to begin with. Your mind certainly helped to get you there — just as everything else in your make-up helped. And a million other factors to boot.

So guilt simply doesn't figure. Maybe sometimes you think, "Boy, if I had cancer, people would be nicer to me. I'll just grow a little tumour, then people will pay attention / my husband will love me more / my children will do more chores around the house / my boss will give me a raise / no one will mind if I stay in bed in the mornings / somebody else will do the carpool." Then, if you really do get sick, you probably would have a major guilt problem. But that is not at all what Siegel, Simonton, Chopra, Dosdall *et al.* are talking about. The difference here is as between a pop magazine misanalysis of a scientific breakthrough —

Mind/Body Medicine: Dealing with the Guilt

"Water remembers!" — and a thoughtful study of a recent experiment concerning cellular memory in water.

Every practising doctor has seen mind-body connections, whether they accept them or not. Placebo therapy is a fascinating example of how some patients respond to a physical "cure" as long as the mind believes. It is a form of faith healing. There are numerous studies of patients responding to sugar pills which they think are medication. The power of the mind convinces the body that it is receiving chemical help. But most doctors, when faced with a patient who has thrown off a virulent, terminal cancer, would rather question the original diagnosis than accept the proof of a healthy survivor of a disease that science says can't be survived.

In February 1990 both *Newsweek* and *Time* magazines carried lead stories on studies that indicated a higher survival rate for cancer patients who were part of a support group. These findings could be interpreted in a variety of ways, but all of them underline the presence of something other than the physical cause and effect of the disease as a factor in survival rate.

You don't think yourself sick or better. The semantics buried in that sentence distort the real meaning. The ghost of the memory which lives in the cells creates a pattern. Your mind is your body, and vice versa. To treat one and not the other doesn't make sense. It now appears that cellular "memory" is not limited to brain cells. The cells of the body "remember" the pattern of the whole and renew themselves accordingly. And where does that pattern come from? Aha. Is it the sum of our experiences? Did it come from each of our personal little Big Bangs — at the moment of conception? Was it lying dormant in the DNA waiting to be activated? If so, what activates it? If it was there before, did it come from nothing? From God? And here we are right back at the Giant Questions.

So if Donna had a few days to spare, I could perhaps have answered her question about guilt. It can't be summed up in a neat and tidy little sentence which inadvertently destroys the very point it is postulating.

Thinking yourself well is a worthy battle credo that does not need to be tarnished by its reverse. It is one more weapon in your arsenal to fight cancer; not the only one, maybe it is only a sling-shot alongside the big guns of physical treatment; or maybe it's the other way around. But why reject it just because it might not work?

I am happy to report that there are cracks showing in the united front presented against mind/body medicine by the mainstream Western medical community. The Ontario Regional Cancer Clinic in Ottawa now has four patient therapy groups that teach meditation and relaxation. The HOPE Foundation in Vancouver, established by Claude Dosdall and Moyra Wright, is very active, holding monthly weekend workshops and seminars. It maintains a large library of books and videos on the subject of alternative treatment and has spawned small HOPE groups throughout Canada. And the first segment of Dr. Alastair Cunningham's course, "The Cancer Patient's Self-help Workbook," is now distributed on cassette and paper copy by the Canadian Cancer Society.

-XXIII-

Bernie Siegel: Peace, Love and Jokes

In 1985 *the prestigious* New England Journal of Medicine *launched an editorial rocket designed to blow the whole mind/body connection out of the water. "Our belief in disease as a direct reflection of mental state is largely folklore." A salvo of criticism poured in. "It's as though I had attacked motherhood," the author of the editorial told* The New York Times. *But she wouldn't change her mind. "Using psychology to combat disease," she says, "is 'like doing a rain dance.'"*

John Barber, "Worried Sick"

[Well, ask the Indians. Rain dances often work.]

The Bernie Siegel workshop was an early step for me in this new world of mind medicine. After Jeannie's note propelled me into the writings of Simonton and Siegel, I could only consider it an omen of some sort that two days later I heard that Bernie was holding a workshop, "A Spring Awakening," in a downtown Toronto hotel over a weekend in March. "No room," the organizer said with regret, when I phoned. "It's sold out, but leave me your name and if there are any cancellations I'll let you know."

"Oh rats," I said, relief flooding my voice with insincerity. Good. I had assuaged my nagging conscience, which was screeching, "Do something! Anything! You miserable wimp." Well, I'd phoned, and they didn't want me. It was now totally legitimate to subside into lethargy again. Chemo had me in a

That Other Place

half-nelson, and I viewed an awakening of any sort with trepidation, especially at night, when the courage quota was nil. It was all I could do to face a new day let alone a new experience. Besides, who would go to such a workshop, pay money to go and hear someone tell you to live, to love unconditionally, to feel exceptional by taking control. Probably just a bunch of kooks. Sick kooks. Sick, desperate kooks. Sick, desperate, gullible kooks. Dumb. I could stay at home, read his book again and save the money. Besides, how could anyone do a successful workshop with 250 people?

There was a cancellation, obviously another damn omen, and I went filled with a roil of cynicism and hope. I'm not sure what I was hoping for — I was beyond the stage where I expected anyone to make me well and cancer-free; I guess I was hoping to learn the next best thing — not how to survive cancer, but how to survive living with cancer. Not just survive, but to come back to life again, out from under this inky cloud of an illness that usually kills, sooner than later.

I flew to Toronto via the now-extinct City Express which lands you at Toronto Island, a civilized way of travelling in this era of air travel spent mostly on the ground getting to and from airports. You'd step off the small prop plane, have your bag handed to you by the pilot, climb directly onto the shuttle bus which creeps all of a hundred feet onto the ferry and across the channel to the Royal York Hotel. Bingo, you are in the heart of the city, having skilfully avoided the chaos and bad temper of Pearson airport, and the Orwellian tangle of freeways sprawling in all directions from Highway 401.

In my university days, 401 was the northernmost limit of the city for us; beyond that was beyond the pale. Recently, in a cab from Pearson airport to a meeting in Scarborough, the chatty driver commented that the city was spreading like a cancer. There it was again, Cancer the Bogeyman, now spreading its metaphoric wings in the skies of city planning. I barely refrained from springing to the defence of cancer — you leave cancer out of this, it has a bad enough name already. I was slightly taken aback by my reaction; why was I feeling protective about a disease, for godsake? I felt as if the cab driver were criticizing me — love me, love my cancer. It was about then that I realized it was time to let go. But that was more than a year later.

The night before Siegel's workshop, I stayed with an old friend. We had dinner in her fine little house south of Bloor, at a table under an enormous, powerful painting that covered one wall; it was of a bull in a field of channels, all primary colours, fringed by a row of marsh reeds, a statement of control. My friend and I had not seen each other for a long while — we reminisced, we laughed about our growing-up years at our cottages at "The Aimers" on the Ottawa River. These were the fine golden summers when we were brown and healthy as trouts, when we spent more time in the water than out, when our parents seemed to turn a blind eye to the wildness of our water ways.

Over salmon steak sprinkled with ginger and garlic, and buttery yams, we continued all the conversations that seem to weave us together forever. There was hardly a break although we don't see each other often. The bond of early friendship has kept us comrades through a lot of disparate years. It was the right beginning to the weekend — it had unhooked me from the grinding familiarity of daily treatment, sickness and the constant struggle to fit both into a "normal" work and family day, all the while trying to keep the mask from slipping.

The Primrose Hotel was the venue of the workshop. Uh huh. Another omen? Was this whole direction simply a detour down a garden path? I was prepared to be completely disappointed. I was prepared to be scornful. I was prepared to be a disbeliever. I bristled with defences. They melted away like snow in summer after the first hour.

The meeting place was an ordinary hotel ballroom. The vivid, quilted banners festooning the walls did not hide the dingy brown and orange colour scheme. The origami butterflies hanging on strings didn't camouflage the smoke-grimed ceiling, flaking in spots where water had dripped from hidden pipes. The room hummed with 250 people, packed in, expectant, hopeful, suspicious. I had expected a visibly ailing audience. There were a scattering of wheel chairs, a few obvious wigs, the occasional grey, lifeless visage of chemo, but mainly the audience looked normal. Normal, whatever that meant.

The workshop had been organized by a Toronto group, members of which were the opening act. With packaged joy and cranked up bonhomie, they hugged and beamed congratulations at each other, at all the love they were doling out. One manic woman suffered from terminal simper. She fluttered and galloped around the dais, her wrists bent like broken wings, looking as if she were trying to launch into flight among the paper butterflies and the dripping air conditioning system. When she screeched that we were all little seedlings and exhorted us to stand and wave our arms like growing trees, I sat like a stump with my arms folded. She trilled that we would all be blooming by the end of the weekend, and my stomach lurched. It wasn't entirely from chemo. I wanted to bolt.

But there was a sense of anticipation and good humour in the crowd. Some were obviously lapping all this up, others were tolerant because they knew what was to come. Many of them had been to the public lecture the night before and were already converts.

Then Siegel sauntered in, ordinary, unassuming, smiling, his baldness the only physical attribute to be remarked upon. He discovered that his shiny dome breaks down barriers. He had launched himself into psychotherapy with a razor. This unprepossessing man, was this what all the fuss was about? I waited for him to put a foot wrong. He didn't. Quietly, gently, he disengaged himself from the foofaraw of the silly introductions, fiddled with the lapel mike for which he had no lapel, and began to speak.

His words, like pellets of shock and truth, rounded with humour, fired with self-denigration and real love, riddled my ready cynicism and desire to hold out. He talked. He wove words and anecdotes — no statistics — he described people he knew and their fight with illness. His theme that first morning was, "Look, my friends, we are all going to die. Get used to the idea. Accept it. And stop living your life like a contest, the first prize being immortality." There endeth the first lesson.

Bernie Siegel: Peace, Love and Jokes

What struck me most about Bernie Siegel was his humour. He is a genuinely funny man. His whole body, his gestures, his facial expression radiates a kind of inner joke, suppressed laughter and *good* humour; not once, the whole weekend did he resort to sarcasm or ridicule. He always laughed with.

At the beginning, we were an audience, all of us looking for something that would quell the fever in our lives, looking for peace or sanity or courage. Our quest, Bernie took and gave back to us as love. We were no longer an audience, but a group of individuals then, all feeling, I think, that Siegel was talking directly to each of us. He had transformed that hot, stuffy, tacky, conference room of 250 closely packed people into a small living room of a few close friends. His main message is love, the age-old message clothed in different words. Unconditional love. He talked about God occasionally, but as an individual in his life, not an all-powerful force — "I tried to persuade God to use flash cards," he said in describing the power of symbols and messages in dreams. Or "God gave Moses three stone tablets, not just two, with five commandments on each. The ones I am telling you now, they were the ones on the tablet God dropped."

He pulled ideas and images from all directions, but the underlying theme was love.

I took reams of notes that weekend; but most of the import you will find in his books. He talked about the importance of living in the present, not a shatteringly original concept since almost every religion in the history of the world does too.'"Sufficient unto the day is the evil thereof," etc. But he has a gift of expressing the idea in such a way that it sticks. He described a clock face — four numbers, 1, 2, 3, 4 ... Who Cares? He invented a clock that would just say NOW across its face. You look up at it and exclaim, "Oh, it's now!" He dealt with the agonized reaction of most of us to a diagnosis of cancer, "Why me?" Why not you? Fair enough. That is the only possible response, like the famous question on a logic exam at Oxford, which asked, in its entirety, "Is this a fair question?" One bright light answered, "If this is a fair question, then this is a fair answer." Full stop. I often think with awe of the mind that could come up with such a response. Some of Siegel's precepts are like that answer. So stunningly simple that they are overlooked, or denied because they have been buried in clichés so long, their meaning has disintegrated with familiarity.

He is indeed charismatic, but is that any reason to disregard him, as some people like Donna argue? His detractors criticize that his message is only the medium — himself. He sells the man, they say, as the Answer. It is all public relations. He tells people only what they want to hear. Odd, I didn't particularly want to hear that I was going to die. Just because he charms his way through to an audience, just because he can deliver a message with such humour that it leaves you aching with laughter, are these grounds for rejection of his philosophy? No. Just be glad that the medium delivering the message is such fun.

He gave us homework: write a suicide note; write a love letter to yourself. Try it. Why is it easier to write the suicide note than the love letter? We were to describe what we would do in an all-white room. I listed the following: I would take off my shoes, quick. I would think how I'd paint on the walls — not paint the walls — but paint *on* them, big bursts of flowers and colour. But I wouldn't do it, just think about doing it. I would arrange a vase with a couple of artful flowers, one small painting, minimal, tasteful. Then I'd forget all about it and curl up in a corner with a good book.

The white room apparently represented your life. My responses seemed to indicate that I am a lazy, dutiful, procrastinating escapist. Or maybe they meant that I had my priorities right. Who knows? There was no fixed interpretation; there was no right or wrong response; it was just a mechanism to make you think, to shake the blinders off your mind, to flick you out of circular thinking, let alone lateral thinking. We're not even close to Edward de Bono here.

Siegel provided his own definition of an optimist and a pessimist: an optimist is someone who is a little vague about the facts, is therefore healthier and lives longer; a pessimist has a better grasp of reality, knows better what is going on, and consequently dies younger. He pointed out that reality was simply a collective hunch anyway.

He talked about learning to love yourself; I thought sure, sure, I know about that, let's move on to something new. But when I tried to write the love letter to myself, my toes curled with embarrassment. Even though I knew that no one else would ever see it, I found it an excruciating exercise but another revealing bit of business.

One of the first steps toward establishing respect for yourself, Siegel said, was to recognize the importance of learning to say no, especially if you are sick, to save energy for yourself and for your own healing. You must protect yourself from demands to conserve strength, space, identity. No need to convince me. I was certainly going to do that from now on, I'd sit inside my space and not feel the least bit guilty saying no.

At the end of Saturday, by which time I ached with the desire to be alone in my room just to assimilate the day's ideas and emotions that bubbled out of the collective energy of that room and Siegel himself, I heard myself agreeing to have dinner with a woman from my group. Jeesu, would I never learn?

One session on the weekend had included a drawing exercise — old hat to many people there, new to me. We were to draw ourselves. Each group — we had been divided into "garden plots" of six by the determinedly whimsical organizers — was issued a box of crayons and paper. We drew the pictures before Siegel explained the significance of colour and details. He showed slides of some of his patients' drawings — a dark despairing portrait by a woman who committed suicide two weeks later, an enormous operating table with coils of serpent-like tubes going into the tiny stick figure on the table, drawn by a child with leukemia.

All the pictures in our group were startling in their revelation of feelings and circumstances, a kind of clarification of attitudes. A couple of the people in my group had done this exercise before and knew the significance of the colours; even though their self-portraits glowed with healthy shades, there were all sorts of details that they had not been conscious of putting in, nor had they directed them.

One woman drew herself as a dwarf-like formless shape, with a spine that hung off her left shoulder like a shepherd's crook. In conversation later, she revealed an almost morbid physical self-loathing; she suffered from severe back pain much of the time. Another woman drew herself in a big armchair overwhelmed by a bookcase of knowledge still to be learned about her cancer — lymphoma. Her husband and baby son were tiny figures lurking on the other side of the wall of books; her preoccupation with her disease seemed to separate her from her family.

I grew more and more nervous about showing my picture, which appeared to reveal too much. So much, that my group, in confusion and perhaps in consternation, asked Bernie to analyse it. My body was a battlefield over which the Bad Guys — cancer — and the Good Guys — the white cells and chemo — fight, stumbling back and forth in skirmishes to win the war. In the picture I am nearly non-existent, just a faint pink outline, apparently a camouflage colour. I had completely lost sight of myself in this battle: I was simply the location over which the battle raged. Apparently I hadn't even taken sides.

When Bernie talked about George, his guiding spirit, his alter ego, God, Karma, call him whatever, I nearly leapt out of my skin. He met George first in meditation, a figure in his mind, he thought, perhaps from his unconscious, perhaps from his imagination. However, he went on to tell a spooky story.

One evening, before giving a lecture, he was waiting in the hall outside the school auditorium where he was to speak. An acquaintance passed him but did not linger. Later this same person approached him and apologized for not stopping to talk to him earlier but said that he hadn't wanted to interrupt his conversation with the Indian gentleman. Bernie was nonplussed. He had been waiting alone in the hallway. What did the Indian gentleman look like? he asked. The description fit George exactly, George who was a figment of his own mind.

When he talked about George I recognized my Clyve. I hadn't known about any of this guiding spirit stuff when Clyve appeared in my head, he just simply was there one day, not an Indian swami but a rumpled Roman soldier.

Clyve's bona fides were indeed bona fide. Somehow I had tapped into the Jungian mainstream. What a comforting thought, that my Clyve — who apparently could also be an earlier reincarnation of me, not such a comforting thought — has a sterling pedigree of the collective unconscious informing him. His references check out.

-XXIV-
Clyve

T. [*tumour*]: *Do you think I threaten your existence?*
[*Claude*]: *Of course I do, you asshole.*

Claude Dosdall, *My God, I Thought You'd Died*
(author in conversation with his brain tumour)

Clyve jumped fully formed into my consciousness like Athena from the forehead of Zeus. He resembles the Goddess of Wisdom only in one respect — he wears sandals. His wisdom is cunning and comes from long experience; he is street smart, and yes, he is wise, but not with that grey-bearded guru type of wisdom that demands immediate respect and awe. Clyve sneaks up on you. He is a stocky little character, middle-aged with sandy hair and a deeply lined face, permanently ruddy from the rigours of the elements. His strong muscled legs are slightly bandy, and his feet are almost round, with tiny vulnerable toes that are useless for climbing. He is easily exasperated, full of impatience for those who do not live up to his expectations. But he is fiercely loyal to his friends. Luckily I am one of his friends.

One of Clyve's guises is a white blood cell, the general of the motley army of white cells that surge around inside me searching out cancer cells to demolish. They are not the most organized bunch, I find, but their hearts are in the right place. Clyve has a small encampment on a ledge halfway up the inside of my stomach from where he issues commands to distant appendages on an old field telephone that only works occasionally. When it doesn't, he has to send a runner, who rappels

Clyve

down the cliff-side to take messages to the various battalions stationed in other organs or limbs out of reach of a megaphone.

His style is rough but effective. "You lot, in the western section, Liver, get the lead out, will you? While you've been leaning about on your spears a whole crowd of cancer cells has sprung up on the northern border of the kidney. Get the hell up there before the storm troopers arrive, or you are tail lights, my friends, tail lights."

The Liver battalion pull themselves into ragged formation, armed with rusty spears and the occasional Uzi. They tug their rumpled tunics into place and move off at a run. I'm not sure why they are in Roman dress, smudged white tunics banded with gold, and floppy sandals, that's just the way it is. They don't ride horses, they don't drive tanks. That would be just silly, horses and tanks galloping and rumbling around inside me ...

Clyve has his hands full with this army. They are eager to do a good job, they talk among themselves in brave loud voices about how they are going to clean up the whole territory in no time. But more often than not, they rush off in all directions like the Keystone Cops trailing loose sandals, dropping their spears in their eagerness to find their prey. When the cancer cells see them coming, they slink into crevices watching silently with their evil little eyes out on stalks as the legions stumble past. Clyve booms out a flurry of orders through a rebuilt PA system that echoes throughout my stomach. "Battalion C, get the hell out of the throat, she's just swallowed a mouthful of coffee and you guys are going to be in the drink if you don't move."

He rams his hand through his hair in frustration. "What's wrong with those idiots? Look at them, half of them have just been swept into the acid pool. Keerist. Who recruited this bunch?" He turns to one of his runners, "Go get Dr. Call fast. I think he's up in the right shoulder checking the tumour site. We need him here now."

Dr. On Call was another important figure in my life those days. He and Clyve kept me sane. Dr. Call wears a rumpled white doctor's coat, a stethoscope hangs around his neck always and he wears one of those silver disks on his forehead, like a miner's light. In the murk of a digestive system, it comes in handy. He is taciturn and efficient; his sanguine presence is a perfect foil for Clyve's explosions of frustration. Between them, they keep the White Army going. They never let the army forget that the cancer cells are weak snivelling little runts, evil, malicious, sneaky, unworthy adversaries whose only strength is in their stealth and their ability to reproduce like rabbits.

I often listen in on Clyve's pep talks to the new recruits. He reminds me a little of Henry V on the eve of battle — the scene is all murk and flickering campfires, the soldiers' faces ruddy in the firelight. It is a tough war, and the White Army constantly needs replacement troops. "This is not a picnic," Clyve says, shaking his head in despair at the raw optimism of the newcomers. "This is a battle to the death. Now you are in the front lines, you not only have to spend every waking hour searching out the cancer cells, you must always be on the lookout for the storm troopers. They're our allies in this fight, but sometimes it's hard to remember that. Especially when one of them comes up and clouts you to kingdom come when your back is turned." A snicker runs through the assembled troops. We'd never turn our backs on a storm trooper. Ho ho. Who'd be so dumb.

Clyve rolls his eyes at Dr. Call. "The storm troopers are being sent in to help us in this fight," Clyve continues, his voice tired from having to repeat the same message so often. "But these guys, uh, well, they aren't exactly selective in their targets. They have big guns, the latest fire power, and sometimes, in their enthusiasm, they are just a wee bit careless who they hit. So be on your guard. You hear me?"

"May I add one little caution?" asks Dr. Call.

"Go ahead," Clyve nods.

"For godsake, stay out of the veins on assault days. You haven't got a chance if you are caught in the first barrage. So make my life easier, and yours longer, by obeying orders and remember just why you are here; not to be heroes but to kill cancer cells and stay alive to maintain peace in this benighted country."

Clyve

"Very poetic," Clyve says admiringly, "Couldn't have said it better myself. OK, fall out, you guys. Report to your assigned areas. And battalion T, keep a sharp lookout for an uprising in your area. You have been assigned the tumour area, and we aren't sure that the enemy has been completely cleaned out up there. Good luck. Now beat it."

He turns to Dr. Call. "Well, you think this crew will have enough sense to keep out of the acid at meal times?"

"Who knows. She's not eating a whole lot these days, so maybe they'll be lucky."

"Yah, but it works both ways: if she doesn't eat, neither do they. And as that little fart Napoleon proved to us, an army can't fight on an empty stomach."

"Depends on whose stomach. In this war it's better to fight in one, yes?" Dr. Call smiles archly.

The inside of my stomach is cavernous, with red, dripping, heaving walls. It is dank and foggy in there; the paths up the stomach walls are slippery and steep. Clyve's site of operations has been chosen for its inaccessibility; there are no paths, just rappel ropes and a single makeshift ladder for Clyve. It is on a ledge high enough that the storm trooper onslaught swirls well below; the only real threat is when I am sick and there is a danger of Clyve and his officers being swept up and out the top. That hasn't happened yet.

The storm troopers of course, are chemotherapy, the Big Guns sent in regularly on a giant mopping-up operation. Unfortunately, as Clyve says, they aren't too careful just who they mop up. The White cells, who are fighting on the same side, often get in the line of fire. So it's a kind of balancing act — a Cold War — in which you must accept the propaganda that the storm troopers are the good guys even as you feel and see the havoc they wreak. White cell counts fall, leaving you prey to every flu bug and cold within 100 miles; hair falls out; the lining of the digestive system is raked with defoliant; eyes get sore, bloodshot and supersensitive to sun, wind, light — to life, in fact. The lining of the mouth and lips erupts in sores, the lower back aches with a crippling throb that maybe comes from the beating your kidney is taking or maybe from the liver, or maybe just from a build-up of chemicals affecting the muscles. (Please understand that this particular theory is completely my own, unsubstantiated by medical expertise, just my own body telling me that it is so.) And through all this sabotage you must hang on tight to the belief that chemo is good for you.

Clyve sprang into being during one of my very first attempts at meditation; I had heard of, but not understood at all, the technique of visualization at that time. At Siegel's workshop I discovered that I had inadvertently been using one of the three main guns of alternative medicine. It wasn't enough, though, just to imagine white cells like little Pacmen chomping their way through dumb cancer cells; I needed personalities and a script. Clyve seemed to be simply waiting in the wings all ready to take the lead role. Dr. Call appeared not long after, written in to help Clyve in the battle. I'm not sure that this is the right way to visualize, the way the books say; I'm not sure there is a right way, except the experts do admonish you not to daydream, but to exercise control in meditation. Whether it is right or wrong, it helps me immeasurably. Perhaps Clyve is an alter ego, and it would be very difficult indeed to continue without him. As long as I keep writing the scripts, he's safe; if I lose control, then he and I are both in jeopardy.

One of Clyve's most important jobs, crucial now as little activities become part of the talisman, the necklace of superstitious ritual that wards off the evil spirits — is to go up to my left shoulder and neck to untie the tension. There is a specific spot where I can feel — and visualize — a knot of muscle and nerve that blocks all the energy. I send Clyve up to untie it. In an instant I am relaxed as a rag doll. No, more like one of those old-fashioned dolls with the hooks and elastics and weighted eyes, with the elastics all unstrung.

Susan Sontag cautions against interpreting disease, cancer in particular, in terms of imagery. To mythologize is to empower the disease with an extra destructiveness. She argues for the stripping away of metaphor which adds a dimension of lies and misinterpretation that further sap the sufferer's strength to combat the illness.

For me, metaphor is one of the most powerful ways of fighting cancer. To face its stark reality without any softening of the edges with language, metaphor, visualization, imagery, history is to go onto the battlefield empty-handed and alone. I am using metaphor right now in depicting cancer as an invader against whom I must take up every weapon at my disposal. Clyve, my rumpled Roman *soldier,* leapt unbidden from my subconscious, I guess, to help me in the fight. I did not consciously sit down and invent him. Your helpers are indeed fashioned after your own needs. In his workshop (and in his book) Bernie Siegel described a patient who, as a Quaker, had a problem with the violence of any visualization that actually finished off the dreaded army of cancer cells. His imagery was much more gentle: he stunned his cancer cells, then carted them off one by one, and laid them gently in a pile to be flushed out of his body later. No violence. His own metaphor.

How ever cancer appears to you, it is valuable to be able to mobilize your resources through metaphor or imagery best suited to your particular image of the disease. And it is difficult to deny the depictions down through the ages that have metamorphosed cancer into a demon mythology.

Sontag's study, *Illness as Metaphor*, is a fascinating intellectual exercise that distances the disease, depersonalizes it, demythologizes it. Perhaps this is her own mythology, *her* way of dealing with the demons. Her plea for abandoning the cloak of metaphor is one of the weapons she uses against the spectre of cancer: deal with cancer as an ordinary disease, don't honour it with a special place in history, fiction or poetry that gives it added power — a mystique that is often proof against scientific knowledge. Sontag wants to fight on another battlefield, one on which her awesome intellectual powers are more effective. For others of us though, metaphor and imagery provide a richer battlefield. Perhaps it does offer greater scope for self-deception or may foster misleading, even harmful, myths. But this battlefield, with its landscape of imagining, for me anyway, is an easier one upon which to fight. There are more crevices to hide in, more swirling mists and clinking armour glinting in the moonlight, more firelight before the battle than on the stark plain of intellect.

One must have a tremendous courage to face the unvarnished truth of cancer. It is not just another disease. It will only become so, as did tuberculosis, as did the plague, when a cure is found for it. Or better to say, a cure for them, since there are hundreds of different kinds of cancer. Then we can pack up our myths and imagery, then we can shake our heads in rueful amusement at the silliness of our attempts to deal with the disease. But not yet. Keep your arsenal well stocked; use whatever works, or whatever feels as if it is working. And when breast cancer is brought to its knees by a new antibiotic, a new genetic attitude or a mutant extract of seaweed, then we can throw away our metaphors or transfer them to the new disease waiting in the wings to scourge our world anew.

July 1990

Sylvia and I had a good visit, chattering like old times. A pink-coated volunteer crept into the room, gently, gently interrupting us.

"Is there anything you would like, Sylvia? Anything at all, before I go?" she whispered in a voice dripping with empathy and caring. Her round blue eyes bore into Sylvia's — direct eye contact was important, don't avert your eyes from a patient's, treat them as human beings. Her eyelashes trembled with concern.

"There's lots that I'd like, nothing that I can have," Sylvia answered dryly. "Thank you for asking, though."

"Can I get you anything? A cup of tea, perhaps?" she turned her limpid gaze in my direction. She was a parody of the perfect caregiver.

I was careful not to look at Sylvia as I answered. In fact, there was no way I could wrench my gaze from this woman's half-nelson stare.

When she had slipped quietly from the room, we both snorted with laughter.

"She's been batting those damn eyelashes at me for three days," Sylvia said. "I'm sure she is an ex-nun."

"I guess she means well, but how many patients do you think she has killed with kindness?"

"Maybe that's why they let her loose in here; she frees up some beds. Do you know what she said to me yesterday?" Sylvia was indignant. "She told me that it was OK to cry."

"Oh God, she's read all the books."

"What I did was giggle."

"But Sylvia, giggling is not one of the stages — there's denial, there's anger, there's resignation, I forget what the other one is, but I'm certain it's not giggling."

"In this room it is. Definitely. What does Kübler-Ross know anyway."

I couldn't believe we were talking that way, and yet it was natural and the laughter was real — not the grief-stricken bursts of guilty mirth of a funeral, not the giggles of nervous tension, but the easy, silly laughter of two friends keeping a spectre at bay.

-XXV-
Mind Over Cancer

The conscious mind is the size of a screw on the doorframe of the house of the unconscious.

Ellen Gilchrist, *The Anna Papers*

An undercurrent of the euphoria of Bernie Siegel's workshop stayed with me for months. Vestiges of it are still with me, reinforced by a second one he held in Ottawa a year later. It was shorter, did not have quite the same impact on me, but that was because of where I was in this journey, not because he'd changed. The only difference I could detect was that God was given a bigger role. Not an exclusive Christian God, but God, an omniscient, approachable, caring — and funny — God.

To use that excruciating expression culled from the lexicon of the behavioural sciences, Siegel's message "empowered" me. Makes me sound like a light bulb, I know, but in fact, the image is apt. His energy and messages electrified me. That first seminar gave me tangible tools to fight cancer, as tangible as surgery, chemo and radiation. It was the encouragement to believe that I could do something for myself, not simply respond to things being done to me. I realized that I could use familiar activities, not new skills or experiences forced on me by cancer, but things I have done all my life — writing and imagining.

The weekend reminded me that I was a person with the same old brain that just needed a jump-start. It was a timely reminder, pulling my head above the rising waters of chemo-induced inertia and depression, not to mention the ever-present spectre of the disease itself, lurking behind the miseries of treatment.

About a month later I started an eight-week course with the Ottawa group, Mind Over Cancer, and a four-week course in quilting at a local shop. I know why I did the former, no idea why I did the latter. It added yet another piece of flotsam to a lifetime littered with good intentions and faded enthusiasms.

I have boxes filled with half-made dresses, macramé wall-hangings that peter out after eight inches of tangled rope, sweaters I started knitting for the boys when they were babies, and before I finished one sleeve they were teenagers. (Since I only know one stitch, it is a complicated procedure knitting a sweater — I started at one cuff and knitted up one arm, across the torso and down the other arm, casting on and off like crazy but ultimately knitting on one straight, boring, line.)

Each September for years I used to sign up for night courses; each October I would quietly quit. I managed to attend two lectures of a music appreciation course before my ears fell shut, and four yoga classes at a local high school that I abandoned because they didn't provide the same camaraderie and chat of the three years of yoga I did in Dublin with a small group of friends. There was always a good reason for stopping.

Aerobics classes, tennis lessons, guitar lessons, all faded after a flashy burst from the starting gate. My worst failure was an exercise class at that same high school. Andy and I didn't even manage to stick it out for the first night; we were late, peeked into the gym to see a motley circle of women already flushed with exertion from walking briskly in a circle under the supervision of a strident, super-fit instructor, shouting, "Now ladies, point your toooooes, stretch those feet, now up on tippy-toe ..." Andy and I looked at each other in silent horror and fled. We never went back.

Here I was again; I was going to learn to quilt a curtain for the window in the bathroom at the chalet, a five-foot expanse of glass that stretched the full length of the bathtub. I didn't even want a curtain on the window — it would interfere with the pleasure of lying submerged in hot water watching the trees sway overhead, it would hide the stars, or the billowing rain clouds.

It would also hide the lighted stage of the bathroom from the forest audience which I suppose could occasionally include a human being. Allen thought so; I didn't care, my theory being that if I couldn't see them, they couldn't see me — an attitude that made me lousy at hide-and-seek as a kid. However, I was convinced after a couple of evenings when I had to roll over the edge of the tub and slither into the bedroom on my stomach to avoid attracting the embarrassed attention of neighbours or workmen in the lane below.

The juxtaposition of the two courses emphasized how far into this new country I was, and how far from the old. The evenings at the quilting course were excruciating: I felt sick, looked sick; I *was* sick. The jolly healthy women around the table, all wielding needles with aplomb, totally intimidated me. I hadn't a clue what I was doing, and peeked surreptitiously at the others' work, watching in amazement as the designs and colour came together in beautiful patterns. I felt absolutely alien — to the people, the activity, the conversation.

Over coffee one evening, one of the instructors spoke with scorn about women who signed up for one course and never came back. "They aren't real quilters, they're just dabblers," she sniffed.

I realized then that I had stumbled into a church and quilting was a religion. Oh god, would the high priestess notice that I had patched in a couple of pieces on my curtain by sewing machine at home? I lived in fear of being banished, the epithet, "DABBLER!" ringing in my ears as I slunk toward the door.

During those same weeks I was going to the cancer therapy meetings — where I immediately felt at home, comfortable in the conversation, with the humour, with the people, with the purpose. Later it dawned on me that this was a religion too for some people, a religion of survival.

The first meeting was scary, no question. I had no idea what to expect but was prepared to go only so far in the "sharing" stuff — yes I have cancer, yes I am in treatment, yes I must be looking for something, otherwise mind your own business. "Support people" were invited to come that first evening — what an unfortunate term, conjuring up a row of crooked uprights shoring up a tilt of ramshackle creatures. But what better term for these husbands, wives, children, lovers, friends, brothers, sisters, mothers, fathers whose faces freeze into a mask to keep the worry and dread from showing? Theirs is a double burden, their own emotions which, if they are not saints, must include resentment at being cast in a role for which they never auditioned, as well as all the emotional baggage they carry because of you.

They must walk the fine line between being Pollyanna and getting their heads bitten off for their troubles, and Cassandra, with the same repercussions. On many days there is no fine line, they are damned if they do, damned if they don't. And unless they come down with a bad case of cancer, their ailments always pale in comparison to the Big C, so they can't even grab the occasional sick day for sympathy.

In my life, my family and my friends, both here and from afar, are the reason I have held together. They have kept me alive and kicking and fighting back the whole of this journey. Without them I'd have caved in at stage one. Occasionally, people I have met on this journey have told me about friends who dropped away, unable to handle the pain of their illness; since they did not know what to say they said nothing, their silence another grief for the individual to face. This has not been my experience.

Two friends, neither of whom I had seen for a long time, came from Ireland and Britain at different times that year of misery, "not because I thought you were going to die," one hastened to explain later. They came out of friendship, and they will never know how much their visits and support helped me handle the badness of cancer's early days. Same with friends and family who wrote from afar, hoping for health, offering love, friends who phoned to wish me well, friends who visited and laughed and were not intimidated by the spectre of cancer in the house, workmates of Allen's and mine who sent lovely luxurious pampering gifts, and continued to check in with magazines and books and good wishes, my close friends, who never let any of the lifelines go. And my family, oh my family who just simply kept me afloat with everything they had to give.

Allen came with me that first meeting of Mind Over Cancer. He was as uneasy as I was. Perched on the kindergarten chairs of the school library waiting for the meeting to begin, we wondered how we had ever come to such a pass. Around the circle, we all introduced ourselves and our cancers; some people were far more forthcoming than others. By the end of the two hours though, already there was a bond, which grew stronger each week.

Ours was a second group of Mind Over Cancer. The "alumni," the first group who had started MOC a year earlier, continued to meet weekly, even though they had completed the three 10-week segments of Dr. Cunningham's course. Their friendships had strengthened way beyond the initial commonality of their disease. In our group, three of the 12 who attended that first meeting did not return. One young woman was simply undone by the whole approach — she said that she wanted desperately to be able to talk about her own illness, to share experiences with other people with cancer, but when it came to the cold reality of sitting in a room with 10 other cancer patients, suddenly the disease took on monstrous new dimensions that she couldn't face. It is not an easy step, that first foray into admission and openness.

And each person indeed was exceptional, to use Bernie Siegel's term, one that I am still uncomfortable with — it sounds so self-satisfied. I was struck by the similarity of this approach to that of Frederick von Meiers who set up an organization he called Eternal Values. Its sole purpose appeared to be to collect lots of money from the Beautiful Young — and gullible — People in New York who bought gems from von Meiers at exorbitant prices in order to survive the end of the world. The author of an article on Eternal Values in *Vanity Fair* (March 1990) mentioned that one of the early steps of inculcating people into a cult was to make them feel "exceptional," persuade them to think that they are better than the rest of the hoi polloi because they had taken control, had recognized the greatness of whatever beliefs they were being encouraged to adopt. I guess Donna might lump Bernie Siegel or Carl Simonton or The Wellness Community leaders into the same charlatan class as von Meier. There are a few hundred differences, however. These giants in the field of alternative treatment do not offer false hope, they do not brainwash their followers and they do not gouge their patients for enormous quantities of money. They do encourage patients to feel "exceptional" though because they were willing to go for the long shot, to expend valuable energy in taking control.

It was exhilarating to talk to other people on this same journey, but threatening to meet people with cancer recurrence. I was frightened by others' stories and wondered if I were not taking my own illness seriously enough (a fear expressed by three other people in the group). It was shocking and heartbreaking to listen to real people talk of their pain and struggle, not just people in books, but people who became friends, so many who have died since.

Pamela: "My lymphoma is the treatable kind; I can get better. I can be cured, and I will." She died within six months of making that statement.

Kate: she had a recurrence of lymphatic cancer: two years earlier, she had radiation, now was on chemotherapy. "My hair hasn't fallen out. Probably won't now. But I am afraid to have a shower in case it all washes off." She was the random sample of one that confirmed my theory that treating your hair gently is not a wise idea: brush it, rub it dry, tug at it, and in some weird way this seems to strengthen it. Kate was back in treatment after a year's remission.

Leonard: lung cancer; he still wore the hospital bracelet indicating that his surgery was new, the shock of his diagnosis still reverberating in his speech, his expression, his haunted eyes. He died within weeks of this first meeting.

Lindsay: she had "indolent" lymphoma, the incurable but controllable kind. She radiated vitality and spunk. Later she was to turn her back on treatment for a time, pack up her life and travel, fall in love, grab the moment. She died two years later.

That Other Place

Janine: with breast and ovarian cancer, apparently unrelated to each other, she had run the gamut of treatment. She still had the strength to give so much to the group. With Lindsay, she was the driving force of MOC, the mothering figure for all of us.

Lucy: a beautiful young woman who had had cancer from the age of 15. For years she had not been able to eat or drink, sustained by intravenous feedings. For our Christmas party she made the best chili ever. Her enjoyment of it was vicarious and unresentful. She died four months later after an operation to try and rebuild her throat and stomach.

These are not the real names of the people in the group. The circumstances, the details, although perhaps assigned to different individuals, are. In any self-help group of cancer patients, these same people will be found — fighters and givers. We followed Alastair Cunningham's course, Segment One with a professional "facilitator" — a term that reminded me of Robo Cop. His job was to lead us through the course, listening, guiding gently, all the time watching for the danger signs of overloaded psyches. But it was the interaction among us cancer patients that was the most valuable, the most healing.

During this time I did a lot of meditating — I called it meditation to legitimize what really were just mind games; extended imaginative play. I kept a journal of sorts: "In meditation tonight I set a crew to hack off any cancer cells in my shoulder ..." "Meditation in morning — there is a special peace up here at the lake. Easier to clear the mind — used the third eye route — went into a candle flame which became a huge cave with light streaming in from one spot. The cave resounded with whispers and roars. I guided the healing light through my body but concentrated on right breast, shoulder and upper back — it flowed like flame in a forest fire and burnt up the cancer cells left over from Clyve's round-up. Clyve and Dr. Call were dirty and sweaty and cross — claimed the healing light was part of the greenhouse effect."

"Tried to do journey-to-the-higher-self meditation on the tape X gave me. I didn't go anywhere. Does this mean I have no higher self? The thoughts of the day kept crowding in, derailing the train that was to pick me up and take me to the more exalted reaches. The tape begins with an instruction to think about an area in your life that you need help on, that needs healing. Well, my mind split into a million fragments because there are so many I couldn't keep focused on any one."

"The journaling tape didn't work today: it says to start with 'Today was the day when ...' and record emotions, etc. Since the day hadn't happened yet when I listened to it, my mind went blank. I tried to use it yesterday, but gave up because my day doesn't seem to fit the tape instructions: it says 'picture yourself at breakfast'; I didn't have breakfast. It says 'picture yourself at lunch'; didn't have lunch, had a bowl of cereal at my desk at 11. So right away I think, 'My day needs more structure.' The hell it does."

Some of the books and teachers say there is no right or wrong way to visualize or meditate. Others, the more advanced texts on Eastern meditation, offer more rigid instructions to achieve the meditative state. During those months I eventually evolved a mishmash of relaxation techniques mixed in with imagery, guided meditation and blank meditation — trying to keep the mind erased and clean of thought.

I have no idea whether this activity has hindered the growth of cancer, but it certainly has reduced stress, lowered the worry level, eased physical pain, and caused consternation among family who hear me, apparently alone in the bath, chortling at the antics of the players strutting about in my head.

In his book *Quantum Healing*, Chopra describes real meditation as the fourth dimension. It is an exciting approach to healing: "The point that Archimedes was looking for — a place to stand on and move the world — actually exists. It is inside us, covered up by the fascinating but misleading moving-picture show of the waking state." (p. 188)

To get there, one must go deep, "to contact the hidden blueprint of intelligence," (*Ibid.*) and *to change it*. Only then can visualization of fighting cancer, for example, be strong enough to be effective. Not everyone has the same mental machinery, the same ability to meditate (the avenue by which you can reach this state), just as not everyone has the physical strength to withstand the onslaught of chemo, for example. Is it fair to condemn the alternative route of mind over cancer holus-bolus because it does not work for everyone? No, the same as it is not fair to condemn radiation or chemo because it does not work for everyone. A certain amount of tolerance is necessary here.

"Suspend disbelief," and give it all a chance.

For those first eight or 10 weeks of MOC meetings I was still in chemotherapy; as a result I remember little except that it was all new, and that it was a tremendous comfort to be in a group of fellow travellers working on something for ourselves.

A refrain runs through all the self-help literature, through Simonton, Siegel, LeShan, Cunningham, Benjamin; they all, without exception, emphasize the importance of taking control of your life; in most instances they mean don't allow yourself to become a victim; fight back, don't tug your forelock and bow deeply to every doctor you encounter, but question, read and find the right route for you.

"Cancer patients who participate in their fight for recovery along with their physicians — instead of acting as hopeless, helpless, passive victims of the illness — will improve the quality of their lives and just may enhance the possibility of their recovery." (Benjamin, Introduction) They become victors over the minutes of their lives. If you simply lie down in front of the steamroller that is your illness, I would say that you are exhibiting distinct signs of passivity. Best to face up to the machine and, like the character in the film *A Fish Called Wanda*, shout "Here c-c-c-comes K-K-K-K-Ken and he's going to k-k-k-kill me," laughing hysterically all the while. And maybe, just maybe, your feet won't be trapped in wet cement, and you'll be able to leap out of the way of the roller. Or maybe you will go down before it, only to reappear later in your life, having survived not only the disease but the treatment too. Then you are truly a victor.

This doesn't necessarily mean becoming an Exceptional Patient, nor does it necessarily mean joining a self-help group, meditating four times a day, or drinking carrot juice until you turn orange. It could mean all these, or none. The important thing is that you make the decision, and that is taking control. It seems to me that it is the sense of control, the self-confidence provided by making a choice that is the healing element, not the choice itself.

An 80-year-old woman in Cornwall had a double mastectomy 24 years ago; she had no follow-up treatment, and today is as healthy as a berry, wearing different sizes of bosoms to suit her moods. She is in control. That is the right route for her.

Another woman diagnosed with metastatic breast cancer responded with impatience: "I do not have time to be sick," she said. "I have too much to do." That was 12 years ago. She didn't give cancer the time of day. And although she didn't join a self-help group, and did not meditate, visualize or stop drinking sherry, she took control of her life just as Bernie's Exceptional Patients and The Wellness Community Victors have.

The cancer therapy group was the right route for me. It was also the right move to leave it when I did. A natural break, it was time to move on. A more selfish motivation was the desire to leave the pain of making such good friends only to lose them so quickly, so steadily, to cancer.

-XXVI-
Every Little Thing Helps

Wallis climbed up on the railing and turned his back on the pool. He did not like back dives much — he was looking for an omen. If I do a good one, and war comes, I'll be lucky. He sprang. The world turned over his head — boathouse, the tops of the willows, the blue sky. He unrolled — for a moment there was a most agreeable sensation of falling on perfect balance — he hit the water too straight and shot straight down to the bottom. He swam to the ramp and crawled out.
  "I've cut my foot, dammit."
  That was the trouble with omens — they came out mixed.
        D. K. Findlay, Search for Amelia

Wallis is a character in one of Dad's novels; his semi-successful dive off the balcony of the boat house into the Mississippi below (our Mississippi, not Faulkner's — the one that winds its way through our childhoods and Lanark County) sums up the usual way with omens.

Four years I spent looking for good omens. I still look. In fact, I have always done it. But during the early cancer years I did it with ferocity. I clung to good signs, and the bad omens I bent all out of shape to look like good ones. This is a legacy from my Mum, who would never allow three candles on a table, and my Dad, who punctuated his conversation with quiet knocks on wood.

One I pounced on was the crumbling of the Berlin Wall. What an excitement it was to watch the Iron Curtain lift, the people pouring through first the chinks, then the whole wide open border that had been a barricade that rent a city, a country and a world in two. We watched, enthralled, the film footage of people dancing and cheering and hugging each other, many of them hardly old enough to remember when the wall went up.

I was certainly old enough, but I was still out by about 15 years when I guessed at the year of its construction. 1961. I had guessed 1947. My early years were not ones of shining political awareness. The wall, though, was the most powerful image of the Cold War, the war that informed most of my growing-up years.

The mixed message of this apparently absolutely straightforward, positive image of progress didn't surface immediately, not until the revisionists started to chip away at the euphoria: does the rest of the world really want to risk a unified Germany? And look what was happening to the balance of power in Europe — it was tilting dangerously. And what's more, West Germany was now so busy bolstering the ravaged economy of East Germany, it was withdrawing its capital from other countries. This wasn't how it was supposed to work.

And that's not all: racism in the united Germany was beginning to look suspiciously like the early paranoia of Nazi Germany against the Jews. Maybe Robert Frost had the right idea. Good fences mean good neighbours. Put back the wall. How easy it is to come full circle on an omen.

The week the wall came down was the week that I waited for results of a second bone scan, occasioned by persistent pain in my back — one of the symptoms they tell you to watch out for. I was scared and depressed — flattened by this return to cancerland when I had only just left it.

I had already had X-rays, which did not show any cancer, but did show a spine bristling with "degenerative bone disease." Arthritis. I knew I had it in the neck vertebrae but apparently in less than two years it had spread the length of my spine. The vertebrae in the X-ray looked as if they had all sprouted horns — little teeth of calcium build-up. Bad, yes. But so relieved was I that it wasn't cancer, I treated it as good news, a skewed example of the theory of relativity at work.

That Other Place

A friend with lymphoma told me about a conversation he had with his doctor. He had gone for a scan which detected what appeared to be a new tumour very deep in the groin. The doctor prodded a little and said excitedly, "There's a lot of fluid in this — maybe, just maybe, it's an aneurism!"

He had another camera wheeled in to look at the offending item from another angle. His face fell, and his voice lost excitement, "It isn't a clot — too bad."

After yelling "Whoopie, I've got arthritis!" my euphoria was punctured by a line at the bottom of the reporting letter accompanying the X-ray: "However, a bone scan is more accurate in detecting metastatic cancer."

It was a different scanning machine than last time, at a different hospital. I had the radioactive dye injection again and loafed around the hospital cafeteria waiting for melt-down. This time I could watch the progress of the scan on a little monitor; I appeared on it as a cluster of dots vaguely in the shape of a stick figure; it was not flattering. It was also unreadable. So was the technician. With an inscrutability rivalling a stone, she assured me that the results would be forwarded immediately to the cancer clinic and to my GP.

Ten days later no one had the results; no one had my charts; my oncologist was on sick leave; and the cancer clinics of two hospitals were at each other's throats. One nurse, long on logic, short on brains, told me that since there were no results, I obviously hadn't had the scan yet.

Sweetly, I offered to wring her neck. She agreed to search further. Somehow I had fallen into a no man's land between two cancer clinics, and both their tracking systems lost me. I was like a low-level plane coming in under their radar — and they squabbled with each other about who was to blame.

It took two more weeks to get the results of the scan, and even then it was verbal. Avoid stress, you are instructed. Stress causes cancer. The scan had detected no cancer; just little patches of fury. The crumbling Berlin Wall was a good omen after all.

During this time I also found myself surreptitiously checking my horoscope, something I had never done before. But what

Every Little Thing Helps

was most telling, the first time I leafed to the back of a magazine, I looked under the sign of Cancer. Cancer is not my sign; in those days, just my way of life. Silly how heartened I was to read my horoscope for July, a full year after my last radiation treatment, with no sign of any recurrence. It said, "Somebody turned over an hourglass next to your crib and warned you about what was going to happen when the sand ran out. Guess what: the sand ran out, and you're still alive and well."

Another theme that runs through these years, along with omens and horoscopes — dogs. These creatures provided the remember-the-time stories that stitch the years, the good and bad times into a healthy quilt of memories, as healing as meditation. We had two dogs then. They did nothing that dogs are supposed to do. They were the kind of dogs that would never be chosen for a dog food commercial because a) they wouldn't eat the dog food, b) they would eat the dog food and throw up, and c) they would bite the producer, the client and the actor, not in a mean or vicious way but because one of the dogs, Tobin, was bad tempered and taken to making Statements about his personal space, and the other, Jem, was just plain crazy.

Tobin was an aging Lhasa Apso. He had been aging for several years but neither his blindness nor his deafness seemed to slow him down a whit. He had an endearing little face, until he showed his teeth, which were crowded, crooked and sharp. He showed them a lot. My step-daughter Loranne was the only person who could get him to haul his teeth back inside his mouth. "Tobin, fix your teeth," she'd order. And he would, he'd tuck them back in until he needed them again to bite someone or something, which was fairly often. He also had an itchy-ear condition which caused him to run around, like a scoop, with first one ear, then the other rubbing along the carpet. His blindness had him caroming off the legs of furniture which he would then snap at in fury, convinced that they had attacked him. If the legs belonged to people, he bit them too.

Jem, short for Jeremy, was a mixed breed. Very very mixed. He came from the pound, where Matt selected him — a quivering

That Other Place

tangle of tawny legs and supplicating eyes — over two rooms full of more promising dogs. Matt would not be swayed. The pound official told us that Jem was six months old, was a husky/collie cross, was good with kids and was a smart dog. He lied on all counts.

Jem had been languishing, unchosen, for so long that when we took him out of the kennel, he had forgotten how to walk. This should have been a clue to his brain capacity. His subsequent behaviour told us that someone in the first year — not six months — of his life, before he became our treasure, had been very cruel to him. For his whole life with us, ten years, he still cowered, shivered and curried favour if you so much as looked sideways at him. He would wring his paws like Uriah Heep, and he was the only dog I have ever met who actually hugged. He'd put his front paws around your waist, bend his head into your stomach and hug.

There might have been husky and collie in him. There was also hound, shepherd and perhaps a little deer — he had the doe eyes and double-jointed legs of a fawn. When he ran, his legs seemed to run along beside him, a disconcerting trait.

Tobin and Jem did not believe they were dogs; they didn't know how to hunt (well, Jem hunted flies, but when one of his ferocious snaps actually captured one, he'd spit it out in astonishment); they didn't retrieve balls or sticks; they didn't catch frisbees; their swims consisted of tiny paddling loops off shore and giant soaking shakes on the nearest towel; they chased cats only if the cats ran away, but if they stood their ground, if they so much as hissed once, our two fearless hounds would screech to a stop and pretend a passionate interest in a leaf, a swooping dragonfly, an arresting smell coming from another direction. They were lousy watchdogs and could be trusted to send up the alarm only if a burglar rang the doorbell and warbled, "Anyone home?" They made messes on the rugs, they ate Hershey's cat food (Hershey is our fine disdainful Siamese cat), they got into the garbage; Tobin hid ancient moulding treasures in our bed, neither came when called, both came when they weren't. I built them a beautiful little designer doghouse, an A-frame with cedar siding. Allen was so impressed he said we could rent it out. To small triangular people. I made a separate room for Jem to hide in, and a shelf for Tobin to loll on and look out a tiny window. They never darkened the door of this bijou.

Despite this woeful tale of their inadequacies, their slightly crazed lives have given us far more than proper dogs could. They've given us stories, enough to fill volumes, that make us fall about laughing each time we retell them.

One morning while I was on the phone, a movement in the kitchen caught my eye. A tiny little mouse with enormous ears — a donkey mouse — was creeping across the floor, winding his way through two dogs and a cat, all who yawned and studied their fingernails and noticed nothing. I whispered to Jem, who was closest, to give chase; he jumped up in fright, stared wildly at the ceiling, and tried to escape through the sliding door onto the deck.

The following morning, early, Allen got up to let the dogs out. He flung back to bed, muttering about the kennel we lived in, and the scratching downstairs started again.

"What's that?"

"Can't be Jem or Tobin — I just put them out."

"Maybe there's a racoon down there?" This would not have been unusual. One evening while we were having our supper on the verandah, a racoon was having his in the dining-room, munching on leftover Easter eggs.

There was no racoon this time, but Hershey was down there stalking something, his tail kinked and twitching. I let the dogs back in to join the hunt. Jem and Hershey paced back and forth trying to look competent. Pacing a few steps behind them was that same little mouse that had routed Jem the day before. They finally noticed him when he ran up on the hearth and squeaked at them. I think he waved.

Jem sniffed tentatively, his ears straight up in excitement, and the mouse scampered right up the bridge of his nose until Jem's eyes crossed. Hershey grew bored with the whole business and ambled out onto the deck leaving me and the mouse chasing each other around the living room. Jem put up a great

That Other Place

pretence by searching and snuffing in as distant a corner as he could find and still be in the same house. Tobin sat patiently on the deck, waiting for someone to open the door so he could join the fray. The door was wide open an inch from his nose, which he held as if pressed up against glass.

Jem's fear of loons caused him to dive through the screen door, leaving it in shreds. He chewed off two deck-door handles, gouged the wooden door frames and dinted the brass doorknobs with his teeth in his attempts to escape those loons. One night he tried to hide in the fireplace. The fire burning at the time deterred him only slightly. He just burrowed in alongside it, smouldering gently.

He tried to dig holes in the dining-room rug, to hide in it. One evening, when the loons were at their looniest, crying and calling on the lake, Jem raced into the bathroom and jumped into the tub, which was already occupied by me and my book.

Jem's terror of life took a new twist during my chemo months. Perhaps it was in sympathy with mine. When he was taken out for his nightly walk, he began to skulk along glued to the walker's knee in the open spaces. This is where, you understand, the snipers can get him — the snipers of life I mean, the symbolic horrors that haunt his singed psyche. Then, as soon as he reached cover he'd plunge into the underbrush confident that he was invisible and safe. What he didn't know was that all the shrubs and bushes flailed like demented souls over his head as he scurried along underneath. He wouldn't have lasted long as a guerrilla. He had difficulty, in the end, lasting as a dog. His fear of the dark grew until he no longer would go out by himself, even in the company of Tobin who, I swear, held his paw as they edged out into the forest. Jem abandoned all hope the minute he entered the portals of night, and would run up and down in front of the sensor light at the back of the chalet to keep the light on. Finally, he ended up being afraid of everything, and it was this fear that did him in. He attacked a friend of Sam's when she bent to pat him; his paranoia and a thyroid gland totally out of whack had sent him over the edge. He was contrite and wriggled with remorse right after he had savaged

Every Little Thing Helps

her, but his terror had filled his whole life and transformed him from an eccentric to a dangerous animal. It was a sad and wretched day when Matt and I took him to the vet for the last time.

But Jem and Tobin, whose old age finally caught up to him; Hershey, Snicker, Sam's guinea pig who also happily bit people; and the occasional visit from Chimo, Sue and Seaton's mildly nutty dog, were a theme, a minor counterpoint to the dramatic chords and melancholy passages of my life all the time I was sick and in treatment. They were a constant, a pure and unaffected melody of mostly comic relief, quite untouched by events and emotions around them.

-XXVII-
Hollyhock

Other people's experiences have helped me cope with cancer; perhaps mine will help other cancer sufferers in turn. Rather like a line of people passing buckets of water to put out a fire — the big hoses and firetrucks are surgery, chemotherapy or radiation, but the buckets are the little bursts of empathy and understanding from other cancer sufferers, a shared experience as important in the healing process as medical treatment.

(Author)

The year following chemotherapy and radiation was hung on the stretcher of check-ups, tests and fear of new lumps and inexplicable and persistent pains. It was a coming to terms with living with the spectre of recurrence. There were Mind Over Cancer meetings, weekend workshops, there was getting back into the swing of work and life. There was the drafting of this book — so much to remember. We now know that one of the causes of short-term memory loss is (check one of the following):

- cancer — it also causes long-term memory loss, and in extreme cases terminal memory loss)
- lack of vitamin B
- menopause
- chemotherapy

I seem to have to check all the causes. Uh ... what causes?
The year was a roller coaster.

Hollyhock

There were days when I woke up full of hope, positively reeking with positive thinking — cancer is behind me, I've won the bout and can get on with life. I will be like those women we love to hear about, the ones who had a double mastectomy in 1920 and no one knew until they died in 1985 of old age. My great aunt lived to be 92 and it wasn't until she was laid out for burial that the family discovered that she had had a mastectomy in the bad old days when cancer was a shameful disease. And breast was a bad word. She had told no one.

About six months after I finished radiation, I developed some kind of infection for which the doctor prescribed sulphur drugs. My body reacted as if I were on chemo again, with a low-level nausea that had me whimpering. Sam asked me one morning when I dropped him off at school, "Does this infection have anything to do with cancer, Mum?" His voice was super casual, as if the thought had just struck him.

I started to say, "Not at all, at all," in my best Irish accent, but caught myself in time. Now what do I do. I wanted desperately to reassure him. On the other hand I was not about to hurl defiance at the gods again. So I said cautiously, "I don't think so." And explained to him why I was hedging my bets.

He knows my superstitious nature; in fact he is as paranoid as I am about putting three candles on a table, and instructs me on the proper way of dealing with spilled salt: "No Mum, not with your left hand. You have to throw it with your right hand over your left shoulder." Allen looks on in disbelief at these exchanges ...

Then there were the days that I woke up not so hopeful. I'd catch myself thinking that it would be any day now that I'd get the second diagnosis. Those were — and are — the days when I look up and stare unflinchingly at the Damoclean sword. On good days I either don't choose to look, or the sword is temporarily out for sharpening.

This waiting game goes with the new territory. There was a celebration for Lindsay when she finished her chemotherapy treatment for lymphoma and had been given the all-clear. Toasts were made, champagne was downed with fervour. She

That Other Place

heard herself saying in her thank-you speech, "when the cancer comes back ..." And it did, six weeks later.

I wanted to put a frame on all this, because obviously it wasn't going to fade away. In June of that year I went to a week-long seminar on cancer — it was to be the bookend of the year, a plateau from which to jump into renewed life. It was held at Hollyhock Farm on Cortes Island off the British Columbia coast, a retreat lodge offering workshops ranging from spiritual healing, writing and singing, environmental issues to a Mushroom Conference.

There are only two phones at Hollyhock Farm. One is out in the middle of a grassy parking lot close by a vegetable garden fenced against the deer. Kept at a minimum, messages from the outside world are posted in the lodge entry, taking second place to more important notices of early morning bird walks, late-night star gazing and bodywork sessions.

The founder of Hollyhock dreamt about it long before he ever saw it; the hollyhocks along a wooden fence were a replica of his dreamscape, which puts him in the same school as the founder of Findhorn in Scotland, another magical place that was the result of a spiritual edict. Apparently Findhorn's founder was strolling through the woods one afternoon and felt the hairy arm of Pan suddenly lying across his shoulders. Instead of rocketing into the tree branches with fright, this very sensible fellow had a chat with Pan who apparently said, "Build Findhorn here and all the veggies you grow will be the talk of the world, so huge will they be." Findhorn is indeed famous now for its enormous vegetables as well as its magical spiritual ambience. Hollyhock is Canada's answer to Findhorn.

The title of the workshop, "Self-discovery through Cancer," cooled me a little, smacking as it did of the "Silver Lining" approach to the disease. The workshop was conceived and led by Claude Dosdall. Like Hollyhock's mentor, Claude also had a dream: to create a network of self-help cancer groups across Canada, to link people who had already taken the first steps outside the hallowed confines of traditional medicine in their search for alternative approaches to cancer. His dream included spiritual and experiential exploration beyond the specific techniques of meditation, relaxation and visualization — a "going through" to the deep roots of healing.

Claude knew of what he spoke — and dreamt. In 1977 cancer very nearly killed him. His doctors said first that he had Parkinson's disease, then they decided that his illness was psychosomatic. Later, as Claude put it in his book, *My God I Thought You Had Died*, the same doctors who had decreed that the disease was "all in his head," turned out to be right — a time bomb in the guise of a tumour in the brain. It was then that the doctors gave him a year to live. That was 17 years ago. In those years, Claude went the limit in his exploration of treatments, lifestyle changes, attitudes and beliefs, before finally succumbing to cancer in September 1993.

With the Hollyhock workshop, Claude laid the foundation for a self-help network. Twenty-one people came from all across Canada — from British Columbia, Saskatchewan, Alberta, almost Manitoba (Kenora), Ontario, almost Quebec (Ottawa) and the Maritimes. We were a disparate lot, but with one thing in common — all but one of us had or have cancer.

It took about 10 leisurely hours to drive from Vancouver to Cortes Island, a trip that included three ferry boat rides and, for some of us, a quart of strawberries, a loaf of bread and a superb lunch at the Old House Restaurant in Courtenay. Arriving at Hollyhock was like tumbling into a time warp, a combination of those summer camps of our youth and the 1960s all over again. Two or three people to a cabin or room, shared bathrooms (ours was across a clearing at the edge of an apple orchard in full bloom), and a quarter mile hike to the main lodge for communal meals, after which, we were informed, we do our own dishes, no shoes in the lodge, and the linen is changed every Thursday. We caught on quickly — this was not the Hilton.

As it turned out, the Hilton could not hold a candle to Hollyhock. The ambience of the farm was almost tangible — a secure isolation from the rest of the world, a sense of peace, a spiritual connection with nature — truly a healing place. All of this was supported by glorious weather, clear starlit skies and a full moon rising over the ocean like a beacon on our last night.

That Other Place

Our meeting spot was Raven Hall, a circular one-room lodge on the hillside overlooking the bay. Huge cedars towered over the round skylight dissected into pie-shaped wedges. It became an oasis within an oasis. During our first session we introduced ourselves, explaining briefly why we had come to such a workshop. Our words were hesitant, shy. Most of the people there were dealing with advanced stages of cancer, and most had simply put a lie to statistics. According to statistics, you don't live for 17 years after melanoma, eight years after as many recurrences of breast cancer, five years after liver cancer. One woman had so far survived 45 biopsies as well as the disease itself.

We divided into groups and talked about fear. It was a gentle, comforting exploration. In one session we traced life-sized drawings of our own bodies. Oddly enough they all came out looking much larger than life-size. It was like being in kindergarten again, scrambling around the floor looking for crayons to illustrate the bits and pieces of our lives around the figures.

"I moved over this drawing like a ouija board," one woman said in awe, after watching her picture develop under her crayons and pens.

For the rest of the week, these haunting self-portraits, like spirits pinned up to dry, draped the walls of Raven — a Wayne Gretzky look-alike, a demented Statue of Liberty, a figure exploding into light.

We made masks of our own faces; we did guided meditations; we danced; we sang. One lazy afternoon we "threw the runes"; it was like a rainy day at the cottage, little groups lying and sitting around the floor, murmuring voices, shouts of laughter. We drew angel cards, the spontaneous responses to which ranged from a fervent "Oh shit" to "Yup, that's exactly right." We did deep breathing exercises; we formed the longest cancer-patient tummy train in Canada. And throughout the days and evenings, at meals, on the deck or shore, in our cabins and rooms, we talked, sharing our lives, forging friendships.

There was yoga at 7 a.m. for those who felt the need to start the day as a pretzel. There was a sunrise boat trip to Long Island,

Hollyhock

dawn bird-watching walks and midnight star-gazing sessions. We did guided meditations, which I like; if you can relax enough, let go, it's like watching a movie in your own head that someone else is directing. Although it is your mind that casts it, writes the script, chooses the locations, it seems to come from another source entirely.

One meditation was led by Doris who took us to meet our inner guide — our spiritual warrior. I thought, OK, I'd better not let it be Clyve, let's see if another figure will emerge. Sure enough, at the end of the sloping path through a forest, in a clearing lit only by the light of a campfire, I saw movement through the smoke. A figure emerged, tall, straight, dark with his face hidden by one of those helmets that have a nose guard down the middle but nothing over the mouth or chin. His cloak fell straight from his shoulders to the ground in even folds — red velvet with gold epaulettes. He wore some kind of metallic tunic underneath.

As I walked toward him, he held out an arm and pulled me into the protection of his cloak. I looked up and suddenly there was Clyve, my tousled disorganized soldier who has been with me so long. He gave me three gifts: a pen — a small version of the one he was wearing like a sword, the copper scabbard green with age; the second gift was a small square leatherbound book. When I opened it out fell a torrent of words. The book was hollow, the words loose and tangled. It was up to me to put them together, to find the meaning.

The third gift, not really a gift so much as a promise of later visits, was a small green frog wearing a tiny crown perched on the back of his head. He might even have been waving a cigar. The crown prince, the frog prince. But he didn't want to be kissed into a human prince. He was absolutely content to be a frog. Where do these images come from? Who knows, but they are more fun than summer reruns.

On the last morning we all brought a gift from nature to the group to symbolize what we had gained from our week. Each laid his or her gift in the centre of the room, saying a few words about its meaning. Some were thoughtful, some moving, some

That Other Place

funny. One of the gifts has a place of honour now on my dresser, an old vitamin C bottle half-filled with sand.

"Some of you might think this is just an old bottle filled with sand," Jim said when he presented it to the group. "Well, you would be wrong. Yesterday on the beach I saw a perfect cloven hoof in the sand. That's what's in this bottle. The grains of sand might be a little rearranged but..." Someone wanted to know if the deer print would reform itself when you poured it out, or was it a puzzle that had to be reassembled.

I was stunned: the bottle of sand was my book of words from the guided meditation, an image I had not mentioned to anyone. The message, the pattern, the meaning is there in the sand or the words, as fine a metaphor as they come for this journey. The universal memory or pattern in us all. Anyone who can reassemble it in his or her lifetime wins the prize, the prize of self-understanding.

On the ferry from Cortes on our homeward journey, a shout went up from one of the crew, "Hey, get down from there!"

A figure was perched on top of a ladder going up the side of the boat's superstructure, his blue T-shirt bright against the bluer sky, his aviator sunglasses flashing defiance at the world. He was one of us, "Like stout Cortez when with eagle eyes he stared at the Pacific — and all his men [us] / Looked at each other with a wild surmise —"

"You can't go up there; didn't you see the sign?" yelled the ferryman.

The sign was a hand held up, palm flat and upright: Halt, it indicates to some. But not to our Chris, our own Cortez, who triumphantly pointed out, *there was no slash across it.*

"I thought it meant that you had to use your hands to climb the ladder," he explained.

"I think Chris might be having trouble reintegrating into the real world," commented another Hollyhocker. We all were. But as Chris's exuberant interpretation of the "forbidden" sign showed, reality all depends on how you look at it. The workshop at Cortes had given us all new perceptions to deal with the old realities.

-XXVIII-

The Dragon Slayers

When we lose our innocence — when we start feeling the weight of the atmosphere and learn that there's death in the pot — we take leave of our senses. Only children can hear the song of the male house mouse. Only children keep their eyes open.

Annie Dillard, *Pilgrim at Tinker Creek*

In the *Globe and Mail*'s Fifth Column (July 1990), Nola Seymoar wrote about how her goddaughter was coping with cancer — not her own, but her mother's. It was a moving account, quoting heavily from the 11-year-old's scribbler in which she was writing a book entitled *Mom and Me*. Her mother had survived four surgeries and chemotherapy in the last two years, and continued to exude vitality and strength in her battle with a virulent cancer.

Her daughter wrote:

Usually when my Mom feels down or angry she tells us, but last Christmas Mom hardly spoke. She slept a lot and sometimes I could hear her softly crying in her room. I was terrified because I thought my parents were getting a divorce. I couldn't imagine anything worse.

Mom remained quiet for a couple of days and I remained scared, until one night she called me into her room. "I have something to tell you," she said in a sad voice. "I know," I whimpered. "You are getting a divorce." "WHAT?" my mom burst into laughter. "Who told you this?" "You aren't? Then why are you and dad acting so strange? Have I done something wrong? What did I do?"

Mom paused for a moment. "No, you haven't done anything wrong. I found a lump on my breast and I've gone to see the doctor about it. It might be cancer."

I was more than scared now. I was terrified ..."Are you going to die?"

When I read this I flipped right back into the guilt pit, because I had done both — I got a divorce and I got cancer, a real double whammy for my kids.

Seymoar wrote, "When adults are not comfortable with an issue such as cancer we avoid discussing it with our children or even talking about it in front of them. Our silence nurtures their fears."

We do it with the best intentions, believing that we are protecting them from the slings of fortune. We aren't though. In fact we are probably intensifying the pain by compounding it with the terror of the unknown. During the summer that I had mammograms and needle biopsies all giving me the all-clear, I was fairly open about it all, because I was so certain, "99 percent certain" that the lump was benign, and indeed that I was making a big fuss over nothing, trotting off for all these examinations. I didn't realize the effect this was having on the boys until Sam's super-nonchalant question, "Do you have breast cancer?"

This really shocked me because until that moment I hadn't myself thought of it in that way. I had worried about the possibility of the lump being malignant, of course, but had gone no further with it. Later I realized that I had been far more frightened about losing a breast than the cancer that could cause the loss. I guess it was a form of protective thinking.

I told Sam that I did not have breast cancer, that he wasn't to worry. And I believed what I was saying, without a doubt, because I had just received the results of the first needle biopsy — negative.

The Dragon Slayers

When the second biopsy indicated malignancy, one of the hardest things I had to do that whole year was to tell the boys. I tried several times, and couldn't. It was as if by telling them, I was accepting the reality of cancer, the tearing, unfaceable, unendurable possibility of leaving them. I could not stand this thought, I could not bear it. By keeping silent, I was trying to keep cancer out of the realm of certainty. And since I still harboured hopes that the surgeon would operate and find that the lump was benign after all, I wanted to protect them from unnecessary worry. Hell, I wanted to protect them, period.

A couple of nights before my surgery, we were sitting around the supper table. Into a pause in the conversation I said casually, "Hey kids, you know all these tests I've been having? Well it looks as if I have to have an operation on this lump in my breast. They seem to think there is something wrong. But I'm sure it will be OK." God, what a lie.

Silence. The boys looked at their plates.

"When?" Matt finally asked.

"Sunday, and I'll be home by Wednesday. Not long."

"OK."

Suddenly the boys were busy. They jumped up and started clearing the table, without being asked. None of the usual horsing around accompanied the chores. They loaded the dishwasher, wiped the counters, put away the food, all the while determinedly whistling. Their whistles grew shrill, and I wept inside.

During the next year, I tried to tell them what was happening, how I was feeling, but most of the time I hardly knew myself. And I kept remembering that day in the car with Sam: "Do you have breast cancer, Mum?" "No, I do not, love." How would he ever believe me again? I wanted to reassure them while still being honest. The line was usually so fine I couldn't find it.

They didn't talk much about cancer. They didn't ask questions about it, and I should have been more forthcoming. They were watchful and caring, and probably as frightened as I was, as Allen was. I prayed that they were not getting scare stories at school, that neighbourhood gossip, garbled as it usually is, wasn't reaching them.

That Other Place

At Bernie Siegel's workshop he had asked everyone to write a fairy story about their own life. It was part of our homework. On the Sunday morning of that weekend I woke at dawn, took my chemo pills and anti-nausea pills, climbed back into bed and began to write. It is the closest to automatic writing I have ever come; it was as if someone else was sitting up in my chemo-clouded brain dictating the words.

When I got home after that weekend I showed the boys and Allen the story, with trepidation, because after it was finished, I realized that it was written for them. I hadn't been able to find the right words to tell them how much I loved and needed them, but I could apparently find the right words to write.

-XXIX-
Dragon at the Door

Once upon a time, in a winter country full of drifting snow and pine trees, there lived a family in a house with many doors. The younger son was a boy who rarely touched the ground in his journeys from here to there. He flew and careened and jumped with the sheer physical joy of being. The house had to have special windows in the upper walls for his particularly enormous leaps out into and back from his outside life.

The older son was physically calmer, but humming with a matching energy that took a different form. He hurled around inside his head in the same fashion that his brother hurled around the room. He would run up and down the stairs many times before he actually propelled himself through a door; his mind was so busy with thoughts, there was no room for remembering his lunch, his books, his tools for the day.

Then there was the stepfather. Now in a traditional fairy story he would have to be villain, because of his label. But he simply didn't fit the bill. He kept his eyes hooded to keep his feelings from showing, to keep his love from shining through. Inside, he winced at every hurt, grew wide with pride at love; he was the protector of the house with many doors.

And there was the mother, a woman of many directions like her younger son, a woman of many thoughts like her older son, a woman of vulnerability, fierce with love, like her husband.

The house had to have so many doors to allow for the scurried comings and going of this family, to let people in, to let people out, to let the winds and capricious breezes of living blow through. For this family had been through the wars and knew that a house with no doors would more than likely blow

That Other Place

up. They knew because they had lived in houses that had done exactly that.

This fairy tale begins with a dragon. Well, perhaps doesn't begin, but continues with one, a dragon that hauled itself out of the swamps of the past, stirred by who knows what voices and whispers. It sucked its fetid feet out of the slushy mud, tossing its head free of the roots and leaves that had encased its body over the years. It reared up slowly, testing its roar and fiery breath to see that everything was in working order after such a long absence from life. Everything worked: fire belched from his dripping throat, scorching the branches above and melting the dirty ice around his belly. The roar shook the frosted trees and hurled the birds into the next county.

Shaking off the centuries, the dragon slouched out of the icy swamp and swayed into its long journey.

☙❧

"So what's the drill today?" the mother asked, as she packed lunches in the sun.

"I'm off to do awesome back-scratchers and a few daffy ducks on the mountain," the younger son said, balancing along the picture rail under the dining-room ceiling.

The older son looped a long leg over the chair arm, his head dipping and swaying with the jazz that curled out of the stereo. "I'm going to finish four essays, read a novel, pick the winner of the Gold Cup, write a letter to the editor, and go out on the tiles tonight."

"I'm off before dawn to build our new house. It will be finished by dusk," the stepfather answered.

And in the space waiting for the mother to answer her own question, through an open door came a sigh, a faint sound on the wind, not enough for anyone really to hear, although they all paused for an instant, listening to the whisper they couldn't hear yet.

The day took place, and many more like them. And the doors stayed wide open, unmindful of the occasional cold that blew in with all the freedom. But finally the mother started to hear the sound, the scurrying breath that grew a little clearer each day, a little more strident. She would stand at one of the doors, shivering a little, wondering if she should close up the house against whatever was out there.

Too late. The whisper, one morning, exploded into a roar of fiery dragon breath that bellowed through the doors, rocking the house, singeing the furniture and catching the mother in its terrible blast. The dragon had arrived. Too late to shut the doors. Too late to ask where it had come from, and why. Too late to bulldoze the swamp, to stop wearing the amethyst ring. The dragon moved into the house with many doors that banged and swung on their hinges like tired eyelids. And the family edged closer, watching it hold the mother in its scaly claws, helpless.

The stepfather tried to fend it off, to drive the dragon out with sheer willpower, since the big guns didn't work. He prayed and bargained with it. The sons circled the dragon, cast spells and curses, gave it a wide berth while moving closer and closer to their mother.

Some days the dragon breathed its scorched breath throughout the house, sending its muted roar into everyone's head as they tried to get on with life around the dragon who had taken up residence in their midst. Other days the dragon slept, its sodden heaving body barely visible in the corner of a room.

It became fairly evident though, that the dragon had come to stay. He was not about to up and leave of his own accord. This beast was not going to slouch back to the swamp to be unborn again, unbidden. So the quiet battle started. To lull the beast, the mother gave it some of her flesh. Just a morsel or two. Then she started to poison the rest of his food, so that when he chewed on her, he grew weaker.

The stepfather and the sons wove a net, so silently the dragon did not notice. But the mother did, and it gave her strength to poison the dragon with stronger doses, and to inch slowly away from its stinking mouth.

Day by day the net grew: the loops pulled tighter, the ropes thicker. At the same time the family wove a rope, thick as an arm, knotted with the help of others too. And in the darkest longest night of the year, they slipped it under the sleeping dragon's claws and around the mother. At the same time they stealthily spread the net around her, between her and the dragon. And slowly, slowly they pulled, tightening the net so slowly that the dragon didn't notice.

For days and weeks they tugged her out of the maw of the dragon. And the dragon, weakened by poison and inattention, loosened his grip on her. Friends and other family came to the open doors of the house, and the windows, and they all pulled on the net. By summer she was free! The dragon gave her up, not with a bang, but with a whimper of defeat.

He might still be in the house somewhere, a mere wisp of his former self, shrunken and cold, a dust ball in a corner, a tiny lump behind a curtain. Or he may have slithered off to his frozen swamp, his fiery roar dampened to a sooty squeak.

The net loops the house with many doors, ready to catch the dragon if he tries to return, or to catch any other intruders. Because the mother, all the while, perhaps unbeknownst even to herself, was helping to make the knots and forge the loops. The net is always there — sometimes strung taut to catch the flying younger son, to hold and support the older son, to guard the stepfather against the breath of other dragons, to protect the mother from old and new ones.

August 1990

Sylvia died last night. In the end it was a release for her, but not for us — her family and her friends. At her funeral I saved up descriptions of people there so that I could ask her who they were, after. And on the way to the cemetery we lost the cortège — arriving at the country graveyard after everyone had gone. Her grave was marked only by new sod and a tiny temporary paper marker with her name.

Unadorned with flowers or fresh earth, the faint outline in the late summer grass offered no comfort, only finality.

-XXX-
Be Glad You Have Cancer ...?

> "Where am I now?" they would say to her. "Can you tell me where I am?"
> Minna would listen and she would tell them: "here."
> It was the only answer any of them ever understood — and no one else had ever said it to them. Here is where you are: with me.
>
> Timothy Findley, *Stones*

I have yet to see anything actually titled "Be Glad You Have Cancer," but that certainly is a theme in the cancer literature of the more extreme fringes of alternative approaches to treatment. "Ask yourself why did you need your cancer?" earnest psychologists advise the poor quivering patient. The possessive pronoun is like a dagger between the ribs.

"What is so wrong in your life that you need the cataclysm of cancer to get your attention, to start to live right?"

Your head and heart reel under the sandbagging of a cancer diagnosis; then your psyche falters under the stinging jabs of guilt caused by such an approach. For a while there I was fairly certain that if the cancer didn't get me, the guilt would.

This is the direction some cancer patients go in quiet desperation to come to terms with their disease. It is the "if you can't beat 'em, join 'em" syndrome taken to last-resort extremes. You have cancer, right? You've gone through the rough treatment required — surgery, chemo and radiation. And you still have cancer. So what else can you change, what else can you offer in expiation to this cruel god? Your attitude.

Instead of fighting the disease and viewing it as an enemy, an unbidden guest that has reduced your life to ruins, you embrace the demon, announcing to all who will listen — cancer has changed my life, yes, but for the better — it has torn away the trappings, I have entered a new and better reality. So let's hear it for cancer. Hurray! Hurray!

This theme was brilliantly portrayed in an episode on the TV series, "Thirtysomething." One of the main characters, Nancy, has ovarian cancer. As her husband says despairingly, "She's been to the moon," and he feels he can't get her back. She's gone to that other place, a country where other people can't travel with you no matter how close they are. She meets another cancer patient who has a fine madness about her, driven over the edge by her illness and impending death. The rage crackles through her strident claims that she and Nancy are lucky to have cancer — now they can live a real life. Translated, this means abandoning all responsibility, grabbing cancer as an excuse for total selfishness.

She tries to pull Nancy into her ken with a cockeyed logic, pouring a kind of demented contempt over all Nancy's old values and relationships. When Nancy turns away in fear, crying out, "I can't talk about it now," the other woman says with a clipped despair, "Now is all I have." And in that short sentence, her terror is revealed. It is a stunningly accurate portrayal.

The morning after I saw this episode I caught myself wondering how long it would be before Nancy's cancer came back and killed her. But wait, wait, this is fiction, for goodness' sake. The scriptwriters can bring it back in order to write the character out of the show, or they can relegate her cancer into permanent remission.

So what makes that so different from real life? Each of us has a scriptwriter who can do exactly the same thing — with a flourish of a pen, write us out of our lives. Some people call their scriptwriters God, some call them Fate, some call them Chance. And then there are those who think that they are their own scriptwriters, the scariest concept of all because it carries with it such responsibility — you write yourself into the disease, so just write yourself back out, OK? Not OK.

At Cortes, Claude Dosdall claimed that some people get cancer subconsciously on purpose to open more doors into spirituality, using it as a lever to flip onto another level of consciousness. Well, that's a theory all right, but not one I am about to accept. I think it is hindsight at work.

Underlying all the self-exploration, the layers of searching for the inner self, the spirituality of an illness that sends us scrambling on a one-person crusade to find the Holy Grail of healing — the New Age lexicon defines it as the inner child, the gestalt followers call it Now — under all of this is the one goal — to get better. Not to have the cancer go into remission, not to fight for a year or two more of living, but not to have got it in the first place. To be healthy.

If we were told we were cured forever, many of us would likely leap right off our chargers and wave the crusaders on by to sink happily back into our old lives and our old ways. But some of us wouldn't. Perhaps cancer is the reason we start to search, but then at some stage of the quest, the reason for setting out is no longer as strong as the reason for continuing — the need to accept with peace, the need to understand. E.M. Forster had it right: "... only connect."

Eternity in the moment — such a trite phrase but with such a motherlode of truth. To reach it, first you have to peel off the layers of pop verbiage and facile expression of the idea buried so deep in cottonballs of cliché as to be meaningless. The film *Dead Poets Society* did a fine job. Carpe diem — seize the day. But it is not 'live *for* the day, but *in* the day, and that is what is so hard to keep hold of. Because of its very prevalence in the literature and philosophies and religions of mankind, expressed in different ways, but always the same message, it loses its meaning. It doesn't stick. We should all have it carved into our psyches, but it keeps fading out, growing over with the weeds of the delusion that we are all going to live forever. And that there will be time for everything.

Be Glad You Have Cancer ...?

We miss the obvious buried in the obvious. Focus on the moment, that is where eternity lies. Combined with memory, it gives you a centre and a weave of life rich and textured, a worthy goal.

I have grudgingly to admit that getting cancer has opened doors I might never have opened, doors that led to profound changes and to knowledge I would not have gained otherwise. But I would happily give it all back in exchange for never having got the disease in the first place.

&c.

In the Great Hall of the Museum of Civilization in Hull, there is a replica of a Haida Indian harbour on the Queen Charlotte Islands. It is suggestive rather than representative, with enormous totem poles brooding over a dock against the background of an impenetrable forest. It is a sparse exhibit, impressive in its simplicity; it suits the huge space of the hall.

The seashore after the tide has gone out is depicted, grey sand and rocks, a few dead fish strewn among the flotsam and jetsam, a scattering of clam shells, hanks of seaweed. Nothing more — no collection of the flora and fauna of the islands, just an ordinary seashore. But people stop and look at it for a long time, the way they would never stop on a real seashore.

It is in a museum, with a frame around it, so therefore must be worth studying. Because of its context — a museum — and perhaps because of its artificiality — it distances the viewer into looking at the ordinary with new observant eyes.

The patient watchers are rewarded, just as they would be on a real shore. The split second you turn away, perhaps wondering to yourself why you stopped to look at the display in the first place, a movement catches your eye. Did one of those dead fish twitch? You watch a bit longer but the carcass lies still. This fish is not on a regular timer. You turn away again, convinced it was your imagination. You made it move simply because there had to be something more to this display than the detritus of dead and boring objects washed in by the tide.

That Other Place

It moves again, a flip of the tail, a creature in the last throes of dying.

I didn't see it at first. Sam did, just the way youngsters see more on a real seashore than most adults. They still have the eye, the patience. Other adults were being dragged back to the display by their children. "Il bouge, ça poisson, il bouge, "insists a small child to his mother. She rolls her eyes and strides on to "do" the next exhibit.

When you walk away from the seashore in the Great Hall, it stays with you in a way that a plain tatty old shoreline does not. You have used your child's eye, or maybe an artist's eye, to see; the framework provides the perspective.

By writing about these past years and cancer, I am distancing myself from the reality of it just as this museum seashore was distanced from a real one. The framework of words allows me to step back and watch with enough detachment to observe a little the flotsam that has rolled into my life with the onslaught of cancer.

It doesn't always work. The reality of a life-threatening disease is too powerful to keep contained all the time. But the act of shaping it with words gives me a feeling of control. It's like taming the dragon, dousing its fiery breath and making it sit still enough to catch its image on the page.

You will have noticed by now that this is not a how-to book — how to have cancer, how not to have cancer, how to survive cancer. None of those things. I am standing right up in that boat in the middle of a lightning storm again, but this time instead of announcing defiantly that I do not have breast cancer any more, I am whispering into the outer reaches of the gods' hearing: I have survived cancer *up to this moment*. I am making no claim for "My Way," nor am I claiming victory.

There are two dangers inherent in survival literature: one is that you discount it entirely, thus missing the nuggets buried in the mulch of nonsense; and the other is embracing it too enthusiastically, convinced by the screeds of success stories that cancer is a mere peccadillo to be banished by positive thinking, a bargain with God or a kilo of vitamin C and a glass of liquid lettuce each day.

Be Glad You Have Cancer ...?

In recent years, the shame of having cancer is being shed publicly; any number of people have come out of the cancer closet and admit to the disease, but usually with the corollary that they are not going to die from it, heaven forfend. That is why it is so shocking when public cancer survivors die.

I read an excerpt of Gilda Radner's book in *Redbook*, on a plane trip from Arizona, the same morning that *USA Today* carried the headline announcing her death. The gutsy spirit of her writing was bathed in the sad ironic glare of those headlines. Hearing first of her death, then reading the story of her "survival" within a few hours of each other, threatened the somewhat shaky stability I had achieved over the months since my own treatment.

Gilda Radner's death did not mean that her struggle had been futile, but it did undermine her publisher's claim that she is a cancer survivor. *She* didn't make that claim; she knew better. What she said was, "I can't ever stop and say, 'I beat it. I licked it.'"

The death of another public cancer survivor was even more shocking. Jill Ireland's book *Life Wish* was so positive it rang like a dinner gong with faith and effort and belief that she would beat her cancer for good. Her second book was a different story, laced not only with her own pain but with the horror of her son's heroin addiction. When she died, I realized with dismay that I was angry at her dying because she sort of promised tacitly that she wouldn't. Self-proclaimed cancer survivors lose their impact as role models when they die.

I am being extremely careful to make no pronouncements. I do not want to be an Abernathy, the poor fellow in an old joke that convulsed our callow hearts for years:

The captain of a ship at sea received a telex that the father of Seaman Jones had died. He asked his First Officer to break the news.

The first officer assembled all the crew on the foredeck. They stood at attention in ranks.

"Seaman Jones, step forward," the First Officer ordered over the Tannoy.

That Other Place

"Seaman Jones, your father is dead. Fall back."

Afterwards, the captain admonished the First Officer, "Listen, that was pretty brutal. You should have softened the blow a little."

A few days later the captain received another message, this time that Seaman Abernathy's mother had died. He called the First Officer again and told him to break the news, gently.

The First Officer assembled the crew in ranks at attention, on the foredeck.

"Attention, men," he shouted. "All those whose mothers are alive, take one step forward ... NOT SO FAST, ABERNATHY."

∞

These are a lot of reasons why I am not claiming to be a survivor. There was that hubristic blow of lightning early on my journey before I even knew I was across the border, when I assured Sam that I did not have breast cancer and as I spoke, legions of little cancer cells were falling about with mirth, slapping their knees and nudging each other, "Hooo boy, is she in for a surprise. Who does she think she is, God?! Hey, Murph, what say we make that expedition into a lymph node today? Our breast base camp is pretty well established now, and those clowns still don't know we are here."

The biggest deterrent to shouting victory from the rooftops is the ease with which the apparent end of the journey, on closer inspection, can reveal itself to be a mirage, just like those cool blue lakes Dad and I saw in the desert in Nevada. I remarked on them first.

"That's amazing, look at that water in the middle of nowhere. Are they reservoirs do you think?" thus exhibiting my propensity for being hoodwinked. I come by it honestly because Dad agreed that it was indeed a fine sight, these lakes on the desert sand, and before Allen could rein us in, we had planned a condominium development on their banks, making us all enough money to buy out Las Vegas.

"They aren't lakes; they are mirages," Allen finally got some airspace in our conversation.

"No they aren't — look, you can see where the highway goes across them on a bridge." We were insistent. As the miles passed, with Dad and I smug in our assurance, the lakes receded, the bridge became a raised junction over a shallow sand valley, and our condos teetered on the banks of shining sand. It is a good thing we're not in real estate.

My first mirage winked out the same way, into the sands of radiation, its disappearance foretold on that same holiday, three weeks before I tangled with the Tumour Board and headed off down another stage of my journey.

The last time we had been in Las Vegas, more than a year earlier, and before I knew of my cancer, I had been struck by the number of sick or disabled people in the restaurants and casinos. Elderly couples were there with young adult Down's syndrome children; through the casinos, parents wheeled their teenage children suffering from grotesque crippling illnesses, parking their chairs by the slot machines while they played hard to win the big one, to balance the bad luck in their lives. An inordinate number of middle-aged couples drifted around, the husbands trailing their wives, their faces pulled lopsided, one leg dragging, the giveaway swing of a useless arm pulled across the body as if in protection against another blow of the heart.

These men had been powerhouses in their time — you could see in their sad wasted faces vestiges of that power — CEOs, company presidents, people very much in control — but a stroke had swept all that power and control away. Now, they were hollow men wizened with anger and frustration. It was like Lourdes, all these afflicted souls flocking to Vegas to kneel at the feet of the God of Luck.

This time, the irony enveloped me like fog when we went into the Sahara casino the night of our arrival. I saw all these people with their visible pain, dotted throughout the slot machines and tables and felt I had joined their numbers. My affliction was invisible but at that moment as tangible as it had been when the surgeon said, "It is cancer." I had crossed into that other place I had earlier viewed with pity and distance, and the dangerous certainty that it was a country that I would never have to travel.

Never assume that any distance is too far to cross. And never assume that the island you've found in the swamp will not shift and sink back into the mud. Within four weeks of this celebratory holiday I was back in treatment.

Positive thinking is fine, but I don't want to push it. To stand right up there and tempt fate by saying "I survived cancer" is sort of like saying, "I survived life." It is with you in one form or another forever, not that you go around with a cloud of doom over your head waiting for it to envelop you in sickness and recurrence and death, but that whatever happens, it is a permanent influence in your life.

I am not ending this book with a victory cry. There is only one real end since this is not fiction. I will end this book without digging a fertile patch in which later ironies can grow.

It is enough to say I am here; and here is always the goal, not a milestone to somewhere else.

Selected Bibliography

Barber, John, "Worried Sick," in *Equinox*, September/October 1988.

Benjamin, Harold H., *From Victim to Victor*, The Wellness Community Guide to Fighting for Recovery (New York: Dell Publishing, 1987).

Bergholz, Eleanor, "Under the Shadow of Cancer," *The New York Times Magazine*, December 11, 1988.

Bradley, Jane and Susan Nass, *Nutrition for the Cancer Patient* (Dallas: Nutritional Research Consultants, 1988).

Breast Cancer: Unanswered Questions, Report of the Standing Committee on Health and Welfare, Social Affairs, Seniors and the Status of Women. House of Commons Issue No. 9, June 1992 (available from Canada Communication Group — Publishing, Supply and Services Canada, Ottawa K1A 0S9).

Brohn, Penny, *The Bristol Programme: An Introduction to the holistic therapies practised by the Bristol Cancer Help Centre* (London: Century Paperbacks, 1987).

Buckman, Dr. Robert, *I Don't Know What to Say: How to Support Someone Who is Dying* (Toronto: Key Porter Books, 1988).

Burns, David D., *Feeling Good: The New Mood Therapy* (New York: New American Library, 1981).

Callwood, June, *Twelve Weeks in Spring, The Inspiring Story of Margaret and Her Team* (Toronto: Lester & Orpen Dennys, 1986).

Canadian Breast Cancer Series, *Understanding Breast Cancer* (Winnipeg: YM-YWCA, 1988). (Volume 5 contains a list of Canadian resources related to breast cancer.)

Cunningham, Alastair, *The Cancer Patient's Self-help Workbook* (Toronto: The Ontario Cancer Institute, no date).

Chopra, Deepak, *Quantum Healing: Exploring the Frontiers of Mind/Body Medicine* (New York: Bantam Books, 1989).

Cousins, Norman, *Anatomy of an Illness* (New York: Bantam Books, 1981).

Cousins, Norman, *Head First: The Biology of Hope* (New York: E. P. Dutton, 1989).

Dickson, Anne and Nikki Henrique, *Women on Menopause: A Practical Guide to a Positive Transition* (Rochester, Vermont: Healing Arts Press, 1988).

Dillard, Annie, *Pilgrim at Tinker Creek* (New York: Harper & Row, Publishers, 1974).

Doheny, Kathleen, "Health Special Report," in *First for Women*, Volume 1, Issue 10, October 1989.

Dollinger, Malin, M.D., Ernest H. Rosenbaum, M.D., and Greg Cable, *Everyone's Guide to Cancer Therapy: How Cancer is Diagnosed, Treated, and Managed Day to Day* (Toronto: Somerville House Books, 1991).

Selected Bibliography

Dosdall, Claude and Joanne Broatch, *My God I Thought You'd Died* (Toronto: Seal Books, 1986).

Dunlop, Marilyn, *Understanding Cancer* (Toronto: Irwin Publishing Inc., 1985).

Ferraro, Susan, "You Can't Look Away Anymore: The Anguished Politics of Breast Cancer," in *The New York Times Magazine*, August 15, 1993.

Findlay, D.K., *Search for Amelia* (London: Geoffrey Bles, 1959).

Findlay, D.K., *Now You Are Wise* (Ottawa: PMF Publishing, 1986)

Fine, Judylaine, *Afraid to Ask: A Book About Cancer* (Toronto: Kids Can Press, 1984.)

Gilchrist, Ellen. *The Anna Papers* (New York: Little, Brown and Company, 1988).

Gill, Derek, *Quest: The Life of Elisabeth Kübler-Ross* (New York: Harper & Row, 1980).

Heaney, Seamus, *North*, "Punishment" (London: Faber and Faber, 1975).

Ireland, Jill, *Life Wish* (New York: Jove Books, 1987).

Johnson, Jacquelyn, *Intimacy: Living as a Woman After Cancer* (Toronto: NC Press, 1987).

Lauer, Robert H. and Jeanette C. Lauer, *Watersheds: Mastering Life's Unpredictable Crises* (New York: Ballantine Books, 1988).

Mansfield, Katherine, *Letters to John Middleton Murry, 1913-1822* (London: 1951).

Mansfield, Katherine, *Letters and Journals*, edited by C.K. Stead (London: Allen Lane Penguin Books, 1977).

Meyers, Jeffrey, *Katherine Mansfield, A Biography* (London: Hamish Hamilton, 1978).

O'Leary Cobb, Janine, *Understanding Menopause* (Toronto: Key Porter Books, 1988).

Roberts, Paul William, "Blood Feud," in *Saturday Night,* December 1992

Rubinstein, Renate, *Take It or Leave It: Aspects of Being Ill* (London: Marion Boyars Publishers, 1985.)

Sheehy, Gail, *The Silent Passage, Menopause (*Toronto: Random House, 1992).

Siegel, Bernie, *Peace, Love and Healing: Bodymind Communication & the Path to Self-healing: An Exploration* (New York: Harper & Row, 1989).

Siegel, Bernie, *Love, Medicine & Miracles* (New York: Harper & Row, 1986).

Simonton, O. Carl, Stephanie Matthews-Simonton and James L. Creighton, *Getting Well Again* (New York: Bantam Books, 1984).

Sontag, Susan, *Illness as Metaphor* (New York: Farrar, Straus and Giroux, 1977).

Ward, Philip, *Common Fallacies II, Dictionary of Common Fallacies*, 2nd ed. (Cambridge, U.K.: The Oleander Press, 1980).